O P M

OXFORD PAIN MANAGEMENT LIBRARY

Opioids in
Non-Cancer Pain

Oxford University Press makes no representation, express or implied, that the drug dosages in this book are correct. Readers must therefore always check the product information and clinical procedures with the most up-to-date published product information and data sheets provided by the manufacturers and the most recent codes of conduct and safety regulations. The authors and the publishers do not accept responsibility or legal liability for any errors in the text or for the misuse or misapplication of material in this work.

▶ Except where otherwise stated, drug doses and recommendations are for the non-pregnant adult who is not breast-feeding.

O P M L

OXFORD PAIN MANAGEMENT LIBRARY

Opioids in Non-Cancer Pain

Second Edition

Dr Cathy Stannard

Consultant in Pain Medicine,
Pain Clinic, Macmillan Centre, North Bristol NHS Trust
Frenchay Hospital, Bristol, UK

Dr Michael Coupe

Consultant in Pain Medicine, Anaesthesia, & Intensive Care
Royal United Hospital Bath NHS Trust, Combe Park, Bath, UK

Honorary Clinical Lecturer
University of Bristol, UK

Dr Anthony Pickering

Wellcome Senior Clinical Fellow and
Reader in Neuroscience,
School of Physiology & Pharmacology,
University of Bristol, UK

Honorary Consultant in Anaesthesia & Pain Medicine,
Bristol Royal Infirmary,
University Hospitals Bristol, Bristol, UK

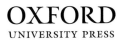

OXFORD
UNIVERSITY PRESS

OXFORD

UNIVERSITY PRESS

Great Clarendon Street, Oxford, OX2 6DP,
United Kingdom

Oxford University Press is a department of the University of Oxford.
It furthers the University's objective of excellence in research, scholarship,
and education by publishing worldwide. Oxford is a registered trade mark of
Oxford University Press in the UK and in certain other countries

© Oxford University Press 2013

The moral rights of the authors have been asserted

First Edition published in 2007

Second Edition published in 2013

Impression: 1

British Library Cataloguing in Publication Data

Data available

ISBN 978–0–19–967807–5

Printed in Great Britain on acid-free paper by
Ashford Colour Press Ltd, Gosport, Hampshire

Oxford University Press makes no representation, express or implied, that the
drug dosages in this book are correct. Readers must therefore always check
the product information and clinical procedures with the most up-to-date
published product information and data sheets provided by the manufacturers
and the most recent codes of conduct and safety regulations. The authors and
the publishers do not accept responsibility or legal liability for any errors in the
text or for the misuse or misapplication of material in this work. Except where
otherwise stated, drug dosages and recommendations are for the non-pregnant
adult who is not breast-feeding.

Links to third party websites are provided by Oxford in good faith and
for information only. Oxford disclaims any responsibility for the materials
contained in any third party website referenced in this work.

Contents

Introduction

Opioids have been used as analgesics for many years. Their use in the management of acute pain related to trauma and surgery is well established. In these circumstances, the duration of symptoms is finite, the therapy is often delivered in the hospital setting, and it can be monitored closely, with side effects managed and optimal dose established. Patients with persistent pain need a pain management plan that brings useful attenuation of symptoms without adverse effects in the short and longer term. Additionally, the management plan must be flexible enough to allow it to be adapted to changes in patient needs and must allow the patient to maintain function physically, socially, psychologically, and, often, vocationally.

Analgesic therapy with opioids might benefit those with persistent symptoms, but efficacy data are discouraging, and concerns regarding the development of problem drug use and the potential for long-term harm highlight the need for careful evaluation of the patient and his/her problems, and a robust and informed continuing surveillance of the therapy.

There is no doubt that patients have been harmed by doctors, either unintentionally or deliberately, as a result of the use of opioids, and the potential for misuse of these drugs has led to an expected scrutiny of prescribing practice. Many doctors are called upon to help patients manage their pain, and a balanced approach to prescribing should prevail. It is important that prescribers are well informed about opioid drugs, the potential benefits of therapy, and the problems that can occur when opioids are used for the treatment of persistent symptoms. In addition, knowledge of legal issues relating to controlled drug prescribing, and an understanding of the background to these, supports responsible and safe prescribing for patients.

There exists a considerable body of data, mostly from the US at the time of writing, which clearly demonstrates that the sustained increase in prescribing of opioids has been paralleled with a growing public health problem of misuse of prescription analgesic drugs. Stakeholder agencies and organizations are working collaboratively to mitigate risk, but the potential for misuse and diversion of opioids should be evaluated and monitored by individual prescribers.

It is not the intention of this book to bring about a general change in the prescribing habits of readers. There are as many different clinical situations as there are patients and therapists, and, to be successful, a management plan has to be a collaborative effort between the stakeholders involved. Our aim in writing this book is to provide the potential opioid prescriber with answers to some questions and, more importantly, to identify the current gaps in our knowledge. We hope this helps inform the, often difficult, decision-making process involved when long-term opioid treatment is being considered.

Chapter 1

Opioids: a brief history

Opioids have been used recreationally and for the treatment of a variety of ailments for six millennia, with poppy seeds and images having been identified in more ancient cultures. The opium poppy *Papaver somniferum* (the only species of poppy used for producing opium) grows in dry conditions in parts of the Middle East and Asia, and it was first cultivated by the Sumerians in Mesopotamia who described opium as 'hul gil', the joy plant. Hardened poppy seeds were scored with a sharp implement at sunset to allow the latex to flow, and the juice was removed from the seeds the following morning and dried into a powder.

There is evidence of opium use by the ancient Egyptians in 1300 BC for the treatment of 'excessive crying in children', and opium-soaked sponges (*spongia somnifera*) were used to facilitate surgery. The term opium was coined in ancient Greece, and the physicians at the time, notably Hippocrates, espoused the use of the drug for a variety of ailments, with effects that have been consistently described by users of the drug ever since. The effect on pain was to make the symptoms less distressing and intrusive. Homer wrote of opium that it was 'a drug that had the power of robbing grief and anger of their sting and banishing all painful memories.'

As medicine advanced in Islamic civilization between the 9th and 16th centuries, the use of opium became more prevalent and was eventually reintroduced to Western Europe by the Swiss physician Paracelsus in the early 16th century as laudanum, a tincture of opium, and in England by the noted physician Thomas Sydenham. Sydenham claimed that opium could be used for the treatment of pain, insomnia, and diarrhoea, and he is said to have commented that, 'among the remedies which it has pleased Almighty God to relieve human suffering, none is so universal and effective as opium.' The virtues of opium were later preached by Sir William Osler, who described it as 'God's own medicine.'

The popularity of opium as a recreational drug inevitably resulted in it becoming a highly tradable commodity. The introduction of tobacco, and the means for smoking it, to China in the 17th century resulted in increasing popularity of smoked opium, and addiction became so prevalent and was perceived as such a moral hazard that several attempts were made to ban the drug. This paved the way for a profitable trade in imported opium to China by the British East India Company, who controlled production and export. Chinese attempts to halt the flow of imported opium led to the confiscation and destruction of huge quantities of opium by the Chinese authorities. The British responded with an unexpected show of naval strength and won the first opium war in 1840 in which Hong Kong was ceded to Britain, and a treaty was signed to open further Chinese ports for the importation of opium. A second opium war followed quickly, and the Chinese were defeated once again.

The subsequent lifting of the Chinese opium ban in an attempt to make imported opium less profitable to the British led to unrestricted trading of opium around the world. Addiction to opium was prevalent, and its miraculous properties espoused by poets and writers. At the beginning of the 19th century, the active alkaloid of opium morphine (named after Morpheus, the Greek god of sleep) was chemically isolated by Serturner in Germany and was marketed for pain relief and for the treatment of opium addiction until widespread morphine use was recognized as generating a more substantial addiction problem. Codeine was isolated in 1832. The development of the hypodermic syringe in 1840 resulted in injection being a popular route of morphine administration for the rapid onset and associated intensity of the opioid experience, and its use by both the oral and subcutaneous route was prevalent in the American Civil War and written reports of opioid dependence appeared.

In the late 19th century, many opium-containing preparations were readily available for purchase by the public. Diacetyl morphine was produced by the German company Bayer in 1898 and marketed as heroin for its antitussive properties and as a cure for morphine addiction—but again, a recognition of its addictive properties resulted in its production being halted in 1913. In the US, concerns about the moral and medical hazards of opioids led first to state-by-state legislation in relation to opium smoking and other opioid products and, subsequently, to the introduction of a tax on opioid and other narcotic use in the US in 1914, which then led to its restriction to medical use for conditions other than addiction and to the eventual ban on all use of heroin in the US in 1924. Two years later, in Britain, the Rolleston Act allowed doctors to prescribe opioids for any indication, including as maintenance treatment for addiction, and only in the 1960s did the practice become restricted to specially trained physicians working in approved centres. In the 1990s, US opioid legislation was relaxed in many states, resulting in the 'epidemic' of prescription drug misuse seen today (see Chapter 14).

Discoveries in opioid pharmacology continued against the backdrop of changing worldwide legislation. The first synthetic opioid pethidine, which is structurally different from morphine, was developed in 1932 since when further phenylpiperidine derivatives, including fentanyl, carfentanil, alfentanil, and sufentanil were manufactured in the early 1970s. Remifentanil was introduced for clinical use in 1990. Opioid antagonists had been identified since the early 20th century, but initial trials were carried out in the 1950s, and clinical studies of naloxone appeared in the 1960s.

The first discovery of opioid receptors in the brain is attributed to Pert and Snyder in 1973, although the notion of specific binding sites for opioids had been hypothesized for some years, and the endogenous ligands were described in publications by Hughes and Kosterlitz in Scotland in the mid-1970s. The myriad physiological roles of these substances continue to be defined. The roles of different receptor subtypes, the effector mechanisms of exogenously administered opioids, and the neurobiology of tolerance dependence and addiction remain an intense focus of research.

Key Reading

Corbett AD, Henderson G, McKnight T, and Paterson SJ (2006). 75 years of opioid research: the exciting but vain quest for the Holy Grail. *British Journal of Pharmacology*, **147** (Suppl 1), S153–62.

Duarte DF (2005). Opium and opioids: a brief history. *Revista Brasileira de Anestesiologia*, **55**, 135–46.

Hughes J (1975a). Isolation of an endogenous compound from the brain with properties similar to morphine. *Brain Research*, **88**, 295–308.

Hughes J (1975b). Search for the endogenous ligand of the opiate receptors. *Neuroscience Research Program Bulletin*, **13**, 55–8.

Pert CB and Snyder S (1973). Opiate receptor: demonstration in nervous tissue. *Science*, **179**, 1011–14.

Chapter 2

Opioid pharmacology

> **Key points**
> - Opioids act through μ, κ, and δ G-protein coupled receptors.
> - The opioid peptides and receptors form an endogenous analgesic system.
> - Opioid analgesics exert their therapeutic action through μ-receptors.
> - Most of the opioid adverse effects are due to μ-receptor activation.
> - The rational choice of opioids is governed by their pharmacokinetic profiles and patient's individual responses to agents.
> - Morphine remains a good starting point to assess the opioid sensitivity of a pain condition.

2.1 Introduction

The introduction of the words 'opium' (late medieval c.1300–1500) and 'opiate' (1543) to the English lexicon predates the first documented use of the term 'analgesia' (1706, *Concise Oxford English Dictionary*). Although all of these terms have ancient Greek roots, it is clear that the concept of analgesia followed after the introduction of opium to the western world. Indeed, we can see that our definition of analgesia flows from the rather miraculous ability of opioids to, selectively, obtund pain while leaving innocuous sensation intact. Opium was used for many centuries before there was any understanding of how it exerted its beneficial effect.

Over the past 50 years, there has been an enormous basic science research effort to understand the mechanisms of action of opiates, with a view to producing better analgesics with fewer side effects and to gain some control over issues such as tolerance and addiction. Although this has produced some spectacular advances in our knowledge (outlined in Section 2.2 Opioid pharmacodynamics), we still have a limited understanding of many aspects of opioid actions and, in particular, in the functioning of the endogenous analgesic system, the role of opioids in reward and addictive behaviours, autonomic control, and also their function in the regulation of the immune system.

2.2 Opioid pharmacodynamics

2.2.1 Pharmacological identification of opioid receptor subtypes

Morphine may be considered the prototype opioid analgesic drug since it was the first component to be extracted from opium. By the 1960s, it was thought that the drug exerted its analgesic effect through an action on receptors within the central nervous system (CNS). However, it took some years before the crucial experiments demonstrated the presence of high affinity, stereo-selective, saturable binding sites in the CNS, indicating that the opioids acted through a specific receptor system.

This identification of the receptors triggered an intense search for the endogenous ligands, culminating in the discovery of a series of peptides, firstly the enkephalins, followed by endorphins and dynorphins, and, more recently, by endomorphins. These peptides are generated from larger precursors (proenkephalin, pro-opiomelanocortin, and prodynorphin) in CNS neurones as well as some circulating leukocytes. Following cleavage, the active peptides are released by an endogenous analgesic system to modulate nociception through an action at opioid receptors (OR). The endomorphins (μ-OR) and the dynorphins (κ-OR) exhibit some selectivity for ORs, but the other endogenous ligands are relatively non-selective. There is no clearly described association between the localization of specific opioid peptides and particular OR classes, and, indeed, it has been difficult to ascribe specific individual functional roles to any of the peptides. This has led to the prevailing belief that they act in concert with in an endogenous analgesic system.

The search for drugs free of the characteristic opioid side effects (i.e. respiratory depression, nausea, addiction) has driven efforts to define the pharmacology of the opioid receptors. Given the diversity seen in the endogenous peptide agonists, it was suggested that there were likely to be subtypes of opioid receptor. The product of this research was the pharmacological definition of mu, delta, and kappa opiate receptors (μ-, δ-, and κ-OR), each with different CNS distributions and potential physiological roles. However, despite the development of receptor-specific opioid agonists (e.g. piperidine derivatives), there is still little evidence that these offer benefits in terms of the reduced incidence of the major side effects (at equianalgesic doses). The chemical structures of commonly used opioid drugs are depicted in Figure 2.1.

The opioid receptor distribution has been mapped (with immunohistochemistry and autoradiography), and they are found at both spinal and supra-spinal levels, with particularly high densities in areas associated with nociceptive processing (e.g. spinal dorsal horn, parabrachial nucleus, periaqueductal grey, thalamus, insular cortex). There is some overlap in the distribution of the ORs, particularly between the μ-OR and κ-OR, but the distribution of δ-OR is quite distinct. Within the nociceptive signalling pathway, there are high densities of μ-OR on the terminals of small diameter primary afferent (C- and Aδ-) fibres but not on larger sensory fibres. This selective distribution may explain why opioids are able to decrease noxious inputs without affecting fine touch or proprioception. They are also located post-synaptically on projection neurones and on spinal interneurones.

2.2.2 Molecular characterization of opioid receptors

The above pharmacological classification has been borne out by the molecular cloning and sequencing of the genes for, first, the δ- and then, in close succession, the κ- and μ-receptors. The opioid receptors are all members of the G-protein coupled receptor (GPCR) super-family (see Figure 2.2).

They show close sequence homology with conserved transmembrane and intracellular loops but with differences in their extracellular loops, and in the C- and N-termini. This is consistent with the known differences in agonist binding and in their coupling to intracellular signalling mechanisms. Interestingly, each of these receptor types appears

Figure 2.1 Structure of common opioids

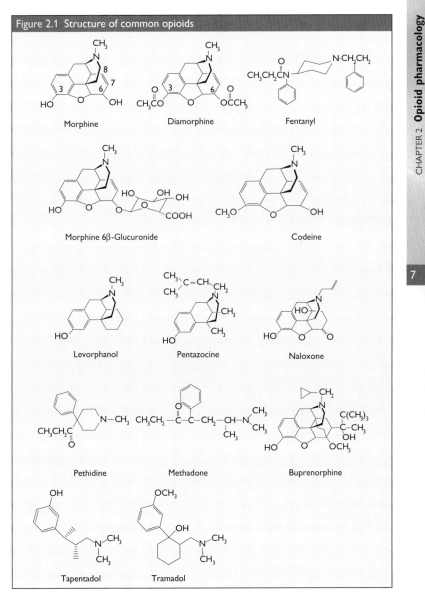

Reprinted from *Opioid receptors and opioid pharmacodynamics*. Davis MP, Pasternak G, Chapter 2, 'Opioid receptors and opioid pharmacodynamics', p. 12, Copyright Oxford University Press, 2005; and reprinted from *Journal of Pharmaceutical and Biomedical Analysis*, 67–68. M. Giorgi, A. Meizler, P. C. Mills, 'Quantification of tapentadol in canine plasma by HPLC with spectrofluorimetric detection: Development and validation of a new methodology', p. 149, Copyright (2012), with permission from Elsevier.

to be coded by single genes; there is no evidence for genes coding subtypes despite the weight of pharmacological evidence (e.g. μ_1 and μ_2). This apparent discrepancy between the pharmacological and molecular data may be explained by either the existence of post-transcriptional splice variants of each OR gene or the effects of receptor oligomerization (e.g. μ-δ dimers).

Detailed knowledge of the sequence of the opiate receptors has lead to extensive studies of the influence of OR polymorphisms in determining pain perception, and the response to surgery or the development of chronic pains (see Chapter 4).

An interesting consequence of the homology sequence screening for subtypes of OR led to the discovery of a receptor with close sequence homology, but no sensitivity, to opioid agonists. This 'orphan' receptor has been renamed opioid receptor-like 1 (ORL_1) and its endogenous ligand identified as nociceptin/orphanin FQ. The role of the ORL_1 in nociception is still being elucidated with evidence for both anti- and pro-nociceptive actions.

Furthermore, this molecular knowledge has permitted some revealing experimental approaches through the use of site-directed mutagenesis to examine the functional organization of the receptor proteins and also to generate 'knock-out' mice deficient in one or more of the opioid receptors. For example, a μ-OR knock-out mouse shows a loss of both analgesic and harmful effects in response to morphine, indicating that the drug's therapeutic and toxic effects are mediated through this one receptor subtype. This may go some way to explain the striking lack of success in the development of opioids devoid of side effects. A similar observation was made in the κ-OR knock-out with the κ-selective ligands. However, the situation is less clear for the δ-OR with, at least, some of the effects of δ-selective agonists being mediated through the μ-OR. These knock-out mice, lacking some (or indeed all) of the ORs, exhibit specific changes (typically hypersensitivity) in their response to acute noxious stimuli, consistent with the concept of an endogenous basal opioidergic tone which exerts an anti-nociceptive effect. This finding is at odds with the observation that the administration of naloxone has no effect on experimental pain thresholds, which had been taken as evidence against the existence of basal opioidergic tone; as yet, this discrepancy is unresolved. The OR knock-out mice also have alterations in their addictive and emotional behaviours, as might be expected.

2.2.3 **Mechanisms of action of opioids**

All opioid receptors couple to pertussis toxin-sensitive, inhibitory G-proteins (G_i and G_o). Receptor activation changes cell excitability through a number of downstream effector mechanisms:

- Increased potassium conductance (producing hyperpolarization)
- Decreased calcium conductance (decreasing calcium influx during action potentials)
- Inhibition of adenylyl cyclase (decreases levels of cAMP)
- Activation of mitogen-activated protein (MAP) kinase
- Activation of phospholipase C (increased inositol triphosphate and glycerol).

These actions decrease cell excitability and reduce the synaptic release of neurotransmitter.

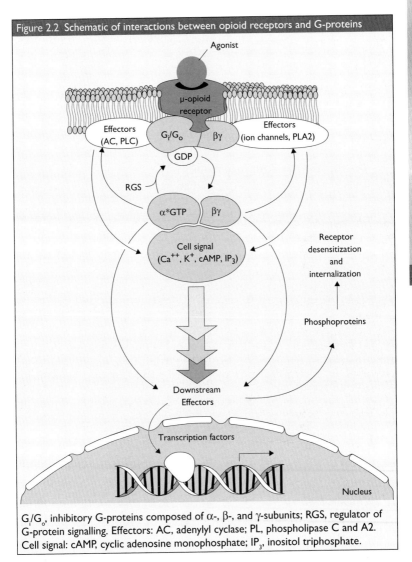

Figure 2.2 Schematic of interactions between opioid receptors and G-proteins

G_i/G_o, inhibitory G-proteins composed of α-, β-, and γ-subunits; RGS, regulator of G-protein signalling. Effectors: AC, adenylyl cyclase; PL, phospholipase C and A2. Cell signal: cAMP, cyclic adenosine monophosphate; IP_3, inositol triphosphate.

Figure 2.2 is reproduced from Davis MP and Pasternak G (2005), Chapter 2, 'Opioid receptors and pharmacodynamics', in MP Davis, P Glare, and J Hardy (eds.). *Opioids in cancer pain*, p. 24, by permission of Oxford University Press.

The overall functional effect of OR activation depends on the subcellular location of the receptors:

• Presynaptic: inhibited neurotransmitter release
• Post-synaptic: decreased excitability of the neurone.

And on the cell type:

• Primary nociceptor afferent terminal: inhibits transmission of noxious information
• Spinal nociresponsive projection neurone: obtunds response to noxious inputs
• Spinal GABAergic inhibitory interneurone: disinhibition through OR-mediated inhibition of GABA release (may be relevant for opioid-induced hyperalgesia).

2.2.4 **Opioid receptor downregulation**

In common with the majority of GPCRs, the ORs show both acute and chronic down-regulation of their function in response to the continued presence of an agonist. Such desensitization at a cellular level is thought to be important in the development of tolerance. The downregulation can occur at a number of levels in the signalling system and also via several different mechanisms at the receptor itself:

• Phosphorylation of receptor domains (PKA, PKC, or βARK)
• Receptor internalization (β-arrestin)
• Increased activity of adenylyl cyclase.

The conventional view is that prolonged application of high-affinity opioid agonists leads inevitably to downregulation of the signalling pathway. However, it has been observed that OR internalization and phosphorylation is agonist-specific, with some agonists, such as morphine, producing much less μ-OR internalization than a selective potent agonist such as DAMGO. These data imply that the coupling of OR to the intracellular machinery is dependent upon the nature of the agonist, opening up the possibility that agonists may be developed that are not associated with the development of tolerance. These experimental approaches have also suggested that receptor internalization is not always synonymous with downregulation as, under some circumstances, it can be a mechanism for the recycling of inactivated cell surface receptors back to their activatable form. There is also evidence that interventions aimed at blocking other neurotransmitter systems (N-methyl-D-aspartate (NMDA) glutamate antagonists and cholecystokinin agonists) can attenuate the development of opioid tolerance.

2.2.5 **Endopeptidases**

The enkephalins are metabolized by metallopeptidases (neutral endopeptidase and aminopeptidase N). These enzymes are thought to terminate the action of opioid peptides within the CNS. These peptidases have been targeted with inhibitors whose effect is to increase the level of enkephalins in the brain, producing so-called enhanced physiological analgesia. The net product is about 40% of the maximal opioid analgesia obtainable using exogenous agonists. The observation that these inhibitors are analgesic indicates that there is a baseline level of endogenous opioid peptide activity that is limited by the action of endopeptidases. It is hoped that this therapeutic approach will be less likely to produce tolerance or dependence than the use of exogenous agonists, although this remains to be tested.

2.3 **Therapeutic actions of opioids**

2.3.1 **Analgesia**
The majority of clinically useful opioid analgesics have their effect through μ-ORs, and, indeed, their major side effects are also mediated through μ-ORs (specifically, respiratory, gastrointestinal, and tolerance or dependence). The therapeutic analgesic effects of opioids are exerted upon several dimensions of pain, both on the sensory and on the affective components, as a result of the euphoria/mood-altering effects. The action of opioids on nociception is mediated at multiple sites, with actions affecting spinal transmission, the relay through the brainstem and thalamus to the cortex, and also actions on the descending control system through the periaqueductal grey and the rostroventomedial medulla. Potent analgesic actions of opioids are seen following spinal administration, and this route of administration does not have mood-altering effects; however, there are strongly synergystic anti-nociceptive effects consequent on additional supra-tentorial administration of opioids. These data indicate that systemically administered opioids act through μ-ORs at a number of different levels of the neuraxis and influence different neural systems to produce the clinically beneficial analgesic effect.

The foregoing, however, does not imply that the other opioid receptors are without functional roles. There is evidence that δ-OR agonists may be useful in man; however, most of the drugs also have actions at the μ-OR in clinically relevant doses. The spinal analgesic efficacy of κ-agonists has been shown, but their systemic use is limited by psychotomimetic side effects. Furthermore, there are some suggestions that systemic κ-agonists oppose the analgesic and mood-altering effects of μ-agonists.

An interesting new insight into opioid analgesia has been triggered by the discovery of peripheral opioid receptors located on nociceptor terminals, and also the synthesis of opioid peptides by immunocytes. These receptors appear to be upregulated by inflammation, and there is good evidence that both systemically and focally administered opioids can exert significant analgesic effects through actions at these receptors. This has led to the pharmaceutical industry exploring the potential for non-CNS penetrant opioid analgesics for inflammatory conditions.

2.3.2 **'Euphoria'**
The mood-altering properties of opioids have attracted much attention, both from a therapeutic perspective and, more pressingly, with a view to understanding dependence and addiction. It is clear that the endogenous opioid peptides play an important role in the 'reward/adaptive behaviour' circuitry within the CNS. There are identified roles for the endogenous opiate receptors and peptides in modulating the release of dopamine within the nucleus accumbens and also in controlling norepinephrine release from the locus coeruleus in a variety of behavioural contexts (presence of a predator or feeding). For example, activation of μ-OR increases the release of dopamine, reinforcing the behaviour, whereas κ-agonists decrease the release of dopamine-producing

aversive behaviours. It appears that the exogenous administration of opioids taps directly into this system and, depending on the context, can produce the characteristic 'high' and the feeling of 'well-being', signifying behavioural reward.

However, it should be emphasized that there is evidence of 'dual' opioid receptor pharmacology whence the functional effect of agonist administration is state-dependent. Thus, a given dose of opioids administered to a patient with pain will produce less respiratory depression/nausea/sedation when compared to a matched control subject without pain. Thus, opioids actually have a wider therapeutic window in pain patients than might be predicted from studies of healthy controls. Indeed, the analgesic effects of opioids are relatively subtle when examined in control subjects responding to evoked experimental pain and are much more easily demonstrated in pain patients. This state dependency of the functional response to opioids may also provide insight into the phenomenon of addiction to prescribed opioids for pain relief.

2.3.3 Other effects of opioids

The original medieval indications for the use of opium and laudanum included antitussive and antidiarrhoeal actions. The antitussive action of opioids (typically, codeine and hydrocodone) is achieved with doses that are sub-analgesic, and they are thought to exert their actions on the cough reflex path within the medulla. There is some evidence that these actions are mediated through both non-opioid and opioid receptors. The antidiarrhoeal actions of opioids are consequent on their reduction in bowel motility and are mediated predominantly in the periphery. Hence, peripherally active opioids (with limited CNS penetration), such as loperamide, are employed.

2.4 Side effects of opioids

(See also Chapter 7.)

The troublesome and apparently obligate nature of the side effects of opioids has driven much of the research effort in the opioid field and has been responsible for some imaginative clinical protocols for drug administration. Most of the significant side effects are predictable consequences of μ-OR activation. The dual pharmacology of opioids mentioned earlier means that these side effects are lessened in patients with pain, but this can rebound if the cause of the pain is abruptly removed, with consequent opioid toxicity.

2.4.1 Respiratory depression

This action is mediated through actions of opioids on the ponto-medullary respiratory centres. There is a suppression of the respiratory rhythm (producing alteration of pattern; reductions in respiratory rate and, subsequently, of tidal volume) and also depression of the central chemoreflex function that obtunds the ventilatory response to increases in arterial pCO_2. This action of opioids is sufficiently powerful to produce complete apnoea and provoke respiratory arrest. Sedation or clouding of consciousness will typically precede or accompany the development of significant respiratory depression. A degree of tolerance to respiratory depression develops with chronic consumption (although even opiate-maintained subjects exhibit significant blunting of their central chemoreflex). This tolerance is reversed rapidly on discontinuation of opioids, a factor that may account for the high incidence of respiratory arrest seen in relapsing addicts, following a period of abstinence after incarceration.

Long efforts to produce opiates with less potential for respiratory depression have been largely unsuccessful. Although the mixed partial agonist/antagonist action of buprenorphine has been suggested to put a ceiling on the degree of respiratory depression (unlike the analgesic action), deaths have been reported from respiratory arrest following buprenorphine overdose, and buprenorphine is relatively resistant to reversal with naloxone. It is noteworthy that, in chronic use, there are some data to suggest that buprenorphine may be safer in opiate maintenance programmes than methadone. Similar arguments about reduced respiratory depression are leveraged about tramadol, but this is likely due to the partial agonist action of the drug at the μ-OR.

Although the respiratory depression associated with opiate overdose can usually be acutely reversed with naloxone, this will antagonize any analgesic effects so cannot be used as a chronic preventative strategy. There are some interesting data now emerging on the use of alternative pharmacological strategies to reverse opioid-induced depression of the respiratory centres while maintaining the analgesic actions. Based on animal studies, several strategies, using 5-HT agonists to reverse the respiratory depressant effects of opioids, have been proposed. There are some supportive human anecdotal reports from extreme cases of respiratory depression, but controlled studies in volunteers have, so far, failed to replicate the reversal of opioid-induced respiratory depression with 5-HT_{1a} and 5-HT_4 agonists. Another area of interest is in the AMPAkines, molecules that potentiate the action of glutamate at AMPA receptors. These receptors are involved in respiratory pattern generation and AMPAkines have been shown in rodent studies to compensate opiate-induced respiratory depression without affecting analgesia. This finding has been replicated in human phase II studies, and phase III trials are now being considered.

2.4.2 **Nausea and vomiting**

The use of opioids is associated with high incidence of nausea and vomiting. These effects are mediated both peripherally, through gastric stasis, and centrally, in the medulla, with actions on the chemoreceptor trigger zone and also on the vomiting centre. This action is worst on initiation of therapy, and the development of tolerance is common. Thus, the prophylactic use of anti-emetics is often indicated on initiation of opioid therapy.

2.4.3 **Constipation**

Constipation can be one of the most troublesome side effects experienced by patients on long-term opioid therapy. This is because significant tolerance to opioids does not develop within the gastrointestinal (GI) tract, in contrast with the other opioid effects. Although the predominant action is mediated by peripheral opioid receptors on the enteric plexus, the neuraxial administration of opioids also diminishes GI motility, presumably by obtunding the autonomic outflow to the gut.

The frequency and severity of constipation clearly limit the long-term utility of systemic opiates for many patients. This has led to guidance advocating the routine prescription of stimulant laxatives (often in combination with softening agents such as docusate) with any opiate prescription to pre-empt the development of constipation.

This strategy can halve the incidence of constipation, but this still leaves a significant ongoing burden of GI problems.

A different approach has been taken with the introduction of a number of peripherally restricted or non-CNS penetrant opioid antagonists to be used in combination with systemic opioids. This is based on the principle that the opiate-induced constipation arises from receptors in the gut and that the analgesic actions of opiates are mediated within the CNS. Although there is evidence for central constipating and peripheral analgesic actions of opiates, it does appear that there is a potentially useful therapeutic window. The non-centrally penetrant opiate antagonist methylnaltrexone has been licensed for use in palliative care practice in the treatment of opioid-induced constipation. However, as it is administered by intermittent subcutaneous infusion, it is less suitable for use in chronic non-malignant pain. Several formulations of oral naloxone (alone and in combination) have been introduced, whose actions are largely limited to the gut by poor bioavailability and high first-pass metabolism. Some data suggest that this can reduce opiate-induced constipation while preserving analgesic actions, although the effects are relatively modest, and the cost-benefit analyses do not at present favour widespread adoption of this approach.

2.4.4 **Urinary retention**

Opioid agonists cause urinary retention and urgency by increasing bladder and ureteric sphincter tonus. This is most common after neuraxial administration but is also seen after systemic use. Elderly men are most at risk of problems, but there is also a significant incidence of retention in women.

2.4.5 **Pruritus**

Pruritus can be a troublesome side effect of opioid use. There are both peripheral (histamine release from mast cells) and CNS (μ-OR-mediated) components. Many treatments have been advocated, including anti-histamines, ondansetron, and propofol. Opioid switching (see Chapter 13) may be helpful.

2.4.6 **Confusion, sedation, dysphoria**

Sedation and confusion are common on initiation of opioid treatment, but often tolerance develops over the course of several days. These effects can be minimized by using a tapering increase in the dose of opioid to reach a therapeutic range. Dysphoria is commonly thought of as a κ-OR action but is also very context-sensitive and thus can reflect the patient's emotional status.

2.4.7 **Dependence and addiction**

It is worth noting that there is surprisingly little correspondence between the biological mechanisms of tolerance and dependence, and these, in turn, are completely separate from the phenomena of addiction. The complex relationships between opioids, individual pain patients, and society are discussed extensively in Chapter 14.

2.5 **Pharmacokinetics of opioids**

There are a plethora of clinically used opioid agonists that have been isolated and synthesized over the 200 years following the isolation of morphine in 1806. Over this time, there have been many waves of enthusiastic adoption of new agents, each promising some improved therapeutic profile. However, as most of these drugs exert their major actions through μ-ORs, the most significant differences between the agents are in their pharmacokinetics. It is worth noting that individual patients can have difficulties tolerating a particular opioid, and thus a trial of another may be successful (opioid switching).

2.5.1 Full agonists

Morphine

Morphine comprises around 10% of raw opium and remains the agent to which all other opioids should be compared. The commonest route of administration is oral; however, absorption is variable and often delayed by slow GI transit and uptake. First-pass metabolism by the liver limits bioavailability to around 25% of the total dose. These limitations of oral dosing have promoted the use of intravenous and intramuscular administration, but these are typically limited to hospital inpatient settings. The hydrophilic nature of morphine means that absorption from buccal, transdermal, and even subcutaneous routes of administration is poor. Rectal administration has been used but confers relatively few advantages over the oral route. Thus, the large majority of therapeutic morphine use is via the oral route. Typical dosing regimens include a delayed-release preparation for baseline pain management and a shorter acting preparation for the treatment of breakthrough pain (and for initial dose titration).

Morphine has a half-life of around 2 hours in healthy adults. It undergoes liver metabolism by glucuronidation and renal elimination. The active metabolite morphine-6-glucuronide, which is more potent than morphine and has a longer half-life, can accumulate in renal failure and may be responsible for much of the analgesic action of chronic morphine administration.

Diamorphine (heroin)

Diamorphine was synthesized in 1898 (3,6-diacetyl morphine), and it was hoped that it would have less addictive potential than opium or morphine (sadly, this proved incorrect). It is a pro-drug of the active 6-monoacetyl-morphine, which is metabolized to morphine. The main advantage over morphine is its greater lipid solubility that facilitates administration by the subcutaneous route and also speeds passage across the blood-brain barrier. The lipid solubility is also advantageous after intrathecal administration, as it is avidly taken up by the spinal cord and is thus less likely to ascend to rostral centres.

Methadone

Methadone is a long-acting synthetic opioid that is extensively used in the treatment of heroin addiction and also has an established role in the management of pain in cancer and, increasingly, in persistent pain of non-cancer origin. It has good oral bioavailability, and the peak effects are seen 1–2 hours after an oral dose. It tends to accumulate because of its long half-life of between 15 and 40 hours, making dose titration difficult. It, therefore, tends to be reserved for patients who have already been stabilized on another opioid. It is metabolized by the liver and excreted by the kidneys. Methadone will accumulate in the tissues, and, after discontinuation of the drug, there will be a long washout period with a mild, but prolonged, withdrawal.

Pethidine (meperidine)

Pethidine was discovered inadvertently as a result of a medicinal chemistry search for new anticholinergic agents. It is the father of the phenylpiperidine/piperidine class of opioid drugs (e.g. loperamide/fentanyl). In addition to its action as an opioid, it also has anticholinergic and local anaesthetic properties. It is a μ-OR agonist whose onset of action is faster than morphine and whose duration of action is typically shorter. Thus, some patients appear to find it gives a more pronounced opioid 'rush'. It is extensively hepatically metabolized, and one of the metabolites norpethidine can accumulate (half-life of 15–20 hours), especially with repeated dosing and in the presence of hepatic/renal impairment. This can be significant as it has a proconvulsant action. Consequently, pethidine has declined in popularity as a first-line choice for longer-term analgesia but is still sometimes used in opioid switching, with the aim of reducing side effects associated with alternative opioids.

Fentanyl

Fentanyl is a pure μ-OR agonist, with high lipid solubility and a short duration of action in acute use (because of redistribution). However, on prolonged administration, it accumulates in the tissues and has a half-life of 4 hours. Several formulations take advantage of its great lipid solubility for buccal and transdermal delivery (patches). These are increasingly popular in chronic pain management. The buccal route is used for rapid control of breakthrough pain, and the patches provide a subcutaneous depot for long-term use (the patch is changed every 72 hours). The patches are preferred by some patients but are relatively expensive, and, to date, claims about improved side effect profiles seem to be rather insubstantial. Furthermore, the presence of the subcutaneous depot means that, in the event of an adverse reaction, there is a rather slow fall in fentanyl levels in the blood, potentially complicating management.

Oxycodone

Oxycodone is similar to morphine in many respects but has better oral bioavailability and does not have the complication of active metabolites. It is well suited to chronic oral administration and has both short-acting and sustained-release preparations. There are data indicating that it is effective in the treatment of neuropathic pain, but it is not clear whether this is a drug-specific or rather just a general opioid effect.

Levorphanol

Although levorphanol is currently not commercially available in the UK, there are data supporting its efficacy in neuropathic pain. It is well absorbed from the GI tract, and it is metabolized by the liver and eliminated by the kidneys, with a half-life of 11–14 hours. In addition to its action on opioid receptors, it is also a non-competitive antagonist at NMDA receptors, although it is uncertain whether this action adds to its therapeutic efficacy.

2.5.2 Partial agonists

Buprenorphine

Buprenorphine is a synthetic partial μ-OR agonist and κ-OR antagonist. It was designed to limit the respiratory depression associated with opioid overdose, and, to some extent, this appears to have been successful, as there have been fewer reports of respiratory depression than with full agonists. It is very lipid-soluble, which has facilitated its use as a buccal preparation and transdermal patch (these routes avoid the high first-pass metabolism associated with oral dosing). It is gaining popularity in the treatment of chronic pain and has also been licensed for use as an adjunctive therapy in opioid detoxification. Inactivation is through metabolism by CYP3A4 in the liver, and, therefore, care is needed when co-administering buprenorphine with drugs that induce or inhibit this enzyme (e.g. antifungals, macrolide antibiotics, and anticonvulsants).

Tramadol

Tramadol is a partial µ-OR agonist, with inhibitory actions on norepinephrine re-uptake, and promotes serotonin release. Because of this mixed pharmacological profile, it appears unusual, in that it seems to have a similar efficacy to morphine (limited only by the recommended upper limit on dosing) and yet has a better side effect profile. Respiratory depression appears rare; constipation is less troublesome, and there are fewer reports of addiction and abuse. However, nausea and vomiting, and dizziness are commonly reported and it is dangerous in overdose. Tramadol has excellent oral bioavailability, and similar dosing schedules are used for oral and parenteral administration. Its elimination is dependent on both hepatic and renal actions, and the half-life is around 6 hours. There have been concerns about tramadol lowering seizure threshold, so caution should be exercised when prescribing in epilepsy.

Tapentadol

Tapentadol is a novel opioid analgesic, with synergistic dual modes of action: it is a weak µ-OR agonist and inhibition of norepinephrine re-uptake. Norepinephrine re-uptake inhibition results in activation of inhibitory alpha-2 adrenoreceptors in pain pathways. The µ-opioid-related analgesic effects appear to be more important in models of acute pain, whilst, in models of chronic pain, norepinephrine re-uptake inhibition plays a more important role. Compared to tramadol, a pharmacodynamic relative, tapentadol shows much weaker inhibitory effects on serotonin re-uptake , thus it has fewer side effects (in particular a reduced risk of serotonin syndrome) whilst having a similar analgesic action.

Tapentadol is formulated as a pure stereo-enantiomer and without active metabolites. It is extensively hepatically metabolized by glucuronidation, leading to substantial first-pass metabolism. The inactive metabolites are themselves metabolized by conjugation, and the vast majority (99%) are excreted by the renal system, with an elimination half-life of 4–5 hours. It is supplied as an immediate-release formulation, and a twice-daily sustained-release preparation, with typical total daily doses of 100–400 mg. It has been licensed for use in chronic pain where a strong opioid has failed to provide adequate analgesia. The clinical use of tapentadol in particular conditions (osteoarthritis, back pain, neuropathic pain) will be covered in the relevant chapters.

Codeine

Codeine is often considered a partial µ-OR agonist because of its limited efficacy. This limited efficacy may be a consequence of its variable rate of conversion into morphine by the liver. It is actually a pro-drug of morphine, and variations in patients' genetic phenotype of the metabolic enzyme CYP2D6 make some individuals unable to metabolize codeine into morphine, and thus they gain no analgesic benefit from the drug. However, it is apparent that codeine alone is responsible for its antitussive action, raising the possibility that some of its analgesic effect is mediated independently of its conversion into morphine. Constipation is a frequent problem with regular codeine use.

2.5.3 **Opioid antagonists**

Naloxone

Naloxone is a broad-spectrum OR antagonist, with competitive action at the binding site. It is only centrally effective by parenteral administration because of almost total first-pass liver metabolism after oral dosing. When administered in the absence of exogenous opioids, it has little effect on baseline physiology; however, this situation is altered in the presence of stressors, such as shock, presumably because the endogenous opioid system is already active. Naloxone is used for the treatment of opioid overdose, with an intravenous or intramuscular dose of 0.4–2 mg every 2–3 minutes (to a maximum of 10 mg total), reversing respiratory depression within minutes. Re-narcotization can occur because of naloxone's short half-life of 1 hour, hence patients may require repeated doses or infusions to match the time course of the overdosed agonist (especially with methadone).

Naltrexone

Naltrexone is similar to naloxone but has a longer duration of action. The drug undergoes hepatic metabolism, and the principal metabolite 6-β-naltrexol has some weak antagonist activity, which contributes to the drug's long half-life. The drug is used to prevent relapse in the management of detoxified, previously opioid-dependent individuals.

2.6 **Conclusion**

Opioids remain the mainstay of treatment for moderate to severe pain. They come with a well-recognized side effect profile, including respiratory depression, nausea and vomiting, dependence, and the spectre of addiction. As yet, none of the available drugs have fully demonstrated dissociation of the analgesic benefit from these side effects. It now seems unlikely that this will be achieved through receptor-selective agonists, as most of the beneficial and harmful effects of opioids are mediated through the μ-OR. However, as our basic understanding of the organization of the receptors and their role in the endogenous opioid system improves, it may be possible to identify ways to manipulate the system and avoid or minimize the side effects. In the meantime, gradual opioid titration, use of adjuncts, opioid rotation, and clinical vigilance remain the best ways to maximize the successful use of opioids in practice.

Further Reading

Dahan A, Aarts L, and Smith TW (2010). Incidence, reversal, and prevention of opioid-induced respiratory depression. *Anaesthesiology*, **112**, 226–38.

Davis MP and Pasternak G (2005). Opioid receptors and opioid pharmacodynamics. In: MP Davis, P Glare, and J Hardy, eds. *Opioids in cancer pain*. Oxford University Press, Oxford.

Evans CJ, Keith DE Jr, Morrison H, Magendzo K, and Edwards RH (1992). Cloning of a delta opioid receptor by functional expression. *Science*, **258**, 1952–5.

Fields H (2004). State-dependent opioid control of pain. *Nature Reviews Neuroscience*, **5**, 565–75.

Greenwald MK (2004). Effects of opioid dependence and tobacco use on ventilatory response to progressive hypercapnia. *Pharmacology Biochemistry & Behavior*, **77**, 39–47.

Heinricher MM (2005). Nociceptin/orphanin FQ: pain, stress and neural circuits. *Life Science*, **77**, 3127–32.

Hughes J, Smith TW, Kosterlitz HW, Fothergill LA, Morgan BA, and Morris HR (1975). Identification of two related pentapeptides from the brain with potent opiate agonist activity. *Nature*, **258**, 577–80.

Kieffer BL, Befort K, Gaveriaux-Ruff C, and Hirth CG (1992). The delta-opioid receptor: isolation of a cDNA by expression cloning and pharmacological characterization. *Proceedings of the National Academy of Sciences*, **89**, 12048–52.

Mansour A, Fox CA, Akil H, and Watson SJ (1995). Opioid-receptor mRNA expression in the rat CNS: anatomical and functional implications. *Trends in Neurosciences*, **18**, 22–9.

McNicol ED, Boyce D, Schumann R, and Carr DB (2008). Mu-opioid antagonists for opioid-induced bowel dysfunction. *Cochrane Database of Systematic Reviews*, CD006332.

Manzke T, Guenther U, Ponimaskin EG, Haller M, Dutschmann M, Schwarzacher S *et al.* (2003). 5-HT4(a) receptors avert opioid-induced breathing depression without loss of analgesia. *Science*, **301**, 226–9.

Oertel BG, Felden L, Tran PV, Bradshaw MH, Angst MS, Schmidt H *et al.* (2009). Selective antagonism of opioid-induced ventilatory depression by an Ampakine molecule in humans without loss of opioid analgesia. *Clinical Pharmacology & Therapeutics*, **82**, 204–11.

Pattinson KT (2008). Opioids and the control of respiration. *British Journal of Anaesthesia*, **100**, 747–58.

Pappagallo M (2001). Incidence, prevalence, and management of opioid bowel dysfunction. *American Journal of Surgery*, **182**, 11S–18S.

Pert CB and Snyder SH (1973). Opiate receptor: demonstration in nervous tissue. *Science*, **179**, 1011–14.

Schröder W, Tzschentke TM, Terlinden R, De Vry J, Jahnel U, Christoph T *et al.* (2011). Synergistic interaction between the two mechanisms of action of tapentadol in analgesia. *Journal of Pharmacology and Experimental Therapeutics*, **337**, 312–20.

Schröder W, Vry JD, Tzschentke TM, Jahnel U, and Christoph T (2010). Differential contribution of opioid and noradrenergic mechanisms of tapentadol in rat models of nociceptive and neuropathic pain. *European Journal of Pain*, **14**, 814–21.

Simon EJ, Hiller JM, and Edelman I (1973). Stereospecific binding of the potent narcotic analgesic (3H) Etorphine to rat brain homogenate. *Proceedings of the National Academy of Sciences*, **70**, 1947–9.

Stein C, Schafer M, and Machelska H (2003). Attacking pain at its source: new perspectives on opioids. *Nature Medicine*, **9**, 1003–8.

Terenius L (1973). Characteristics of the 'receptor' for narcotic analgesics in synaptic plasma membrane fraction from rat brain. *Acta Pharmacologica et Toxicologica (Copenh)*, **33**, 377–84.

Wade WE and Spruill WJ (2009). Tapentadol hydrochloride: a centrally acting oral analgesic. *Clinical Therapeutics*, **31**, 2804–18.

Yaksh TL and Noueihed R (1985). The physiology and pharmacology of spinal opiates. *Annual Review of Pharmacology and Toxicology*, **25**, 433–62.

Chapter 3

Opioid actions: insights from imaging

Key points

- The use of radiolabelled opioid ligands has enabled the distribution of receptors to be mapped in health and in some chronic pain conditions.
- Changes in the receptor distribution have been suggested to play a role in the pathology of some chronic pain states and may also be associated with heritable traits such as COMT polymorphism.
- Dynamic assessment of radioligand binding has been used to reveal the engagement of the endogenous opioid system during maintained painful stimulation and during placebo expectation of analgesia.
- Activation of areas, such as the anterior cingulate cortex, appears to be associated with the analgesic effects of exogenous opioids.

3.1 Introduction

Much of our current understanding of the action of both endogenous and exogenous opioids comes from animal work that has been extrapolated to humans. It is clear that there are many similarities between the functional organization of this system in rodents, primates, and man, with similar distributions of ORs and peptides (as indicated from human post-mortem tissue). However, if we are to better understand the role of the opioid system in complex human behaviours, such as pain, reward, stress, and addiction, then we need to explore the functioning system in man *in vivo*. Just such an opportunity has been presented with the development of functional neuroimaging techniques such as radioligand positron emission tomography (PET) and also pharmaco-functional magnetic resonance imaging (pharmaco-f MRI). While the technological and methodological aspects of these approaches are beyond the scope of this book, there are some findings from these studies which have broad implications and merit further discussion.

The development of opioid radioligands, such as [^{11}C]-carfentanil (a selective μ-OR agonist), [^{11}C]- and [^{18}F]-diprenorphine (a broad-spectrum opioid antagonist), and [^{18}F]-cyclofoxy (μ- and κ-OR antagonist), has allowed the distribution of ORs to be mapped in man *in vivo*, using a relatively non-invasive approach. These studies have focused predominantly on supra-tentorial structures, largely for technical reasons, although some attention has been paid, more recently, to brainstem structures such as the periaqueductal grey. This supra-tentorial focus is interesting, as these centres are involved in the emotional and affective dimensions of pain as well as the sensory-discriminative dimension; thus, these findings augment and extend the existing animal data.

3.2 **Opioid receptor distribution**

The ORs have a non-uniform distribution being found in regions associated with pain processing with a predominance in the medial, rather than the lateral, pain pathway. This may indicate that the endogenous opioid system is more involved in modulating the affective and motivational aspects of pain (carried in the medial system) rather than the sensory-discriminative processing that is predominantly coded in the lateral system. This work has been extended to show that there are age- and gender-related differences in opioid binding. The gender differences are interesting, as women show higher densities of OR binding in a number of regions, including the anterior cingulate, prefrontal, parietal, and temporal cortices as well as the amygdala. The receptor density in some of these regions also appears to change with the oestrus cycle and correlates with circulating oestrogen levels, and post-menopausal women show lower opioid binding than age-matched men. These gender differences may go some way to accounting for the observed differences in opioid sensitivity seen in women who seem more sensitive to μ-OR agonists.

Inherited influences on opioid sensitivity and susceptibility (e.g. addiction) have been the focus of much attention. Thus, it is interesting that changes in the μ-OR distribution have been linked to polymorphisms of the catechol-o-methyl transferase (COMT) gene, which metabolizes dopamine and norepinephrine. These polymorphisms, that change function in the catecholaminergic system, are associated with altered μ-OR binding seen in the thalamus, and this correlates with changes in their sensory-affective responses to experimental pain stimuli. This sort of approach may delineate some of the reasons behind the observed variability in the pain experience for patients exposed to similar insults.

3.3 **Site of action of exogenous opioids**

Despite the large body of data on opioids, it is still not certain which particular regions of the brain (especially supra-tentorial areas) are responsible for producing the therapeutic effects of exogenously administered opioids. The use of $H_2^{15}O$ PET and fMRI during opioid administration has shown which areas of the brain have changes in their activity. For example, there are changes in activity in the anterior cingulate cortex (ACC) that seem to be associated with the analgesic action of the opioid. This role of the ACC in mediating opioid analgesia (in addition to the periaqueductal grey) has also been suggested from studies contrasting the blood flow changes of placebo analgesia with those on administration of exogenous opioid.

3.4 **Evoked pain**

An exciting new development has been the ability to link acute changes in binding potential with the release of endogenous opioids. Although there are a number of significant caveats associated with extrapolating from changes in [^{11}C]-carfentanil binding potential to the actual events at the receptor, this approach seems to be providing revealing insights into the operation of the endogenous opioid system. It has been shown that, in response to a persistent noxious stimulation of constant intensity, there is activation of the endogenous opioid system, and that this activation correlates with changes in the sensory and affective dimensions of the pain experienced. Comparable findings have been reported, using a different radioligand, ([^{18}F]-diprenorphine), and heat pain stimulation. The effects of expectation of placebo analgesia have also been shown to involve changes in opioid binding, consistent with activation of the endogenous opioid system in areas such as the rostral anterior cingulate, the dorsolateral prefrontal cortex, the insular cortex, and the nucleus accumbens. This matches well with the observation that placebo analgesia is, at least in part, reversed by naloxone. A further extension of this approach has shown correlations between OR binding potential and individual variations in the response to quantitative sensory testing, e.g. cold pain sensitivity was associated with lower levels of opiate receptors in the insular cortex.

3.5 **Clinical and ongoing pains**

A long-held aspiration in pain research is the ability to image ongoing pain and, although this still remains just an aspiration, several opioid PET studies have revealed interesting glimpses of changes in the endogenous analgesic circuitry in patients with chronic pain. For example, in patients with central post-stroke pain, there are decreases in their opioid binding in areas associated with pain processing, which is not seen in patients with peripheral neuropathic pain, perhaps explaining why their pains are relatively resistant to opioids. Furthermore, imaging patients with chronic pain (rheumatoid arthritis and trigeminal neuralgia) on 'good' and 'bad' days has revealed falls in opioid-binding potential and in pain-processing areas, associated with the ongoing pain.

3.6 **Conclusions**

Functional imaging of the opioid system holds much promise for the future. In particular, the ability to assess the relationship between complex human pain-related behaviours, genetic heritage, and changes in the activation state of the opioid system is likely to be revealing. There are some significant methodological hurdles to overcome before this will be a clinically usable tool, but, in the near future, it is likely to make a significant contribution to our understanding of mechanisms and, hence, to the development of novel analgesic strategies.

Key Reading

Casey KL, Svensson P, Morrow TJ, Raz J, Jone C, and Minoshima S (2000). Selective opiate modulation of nociceptive processing in the human brain. *Journal of Neurophysiology*, **84**, 525–33.

Henriksen G and Willoch F (2008). Imaging of opioid receptors in the central nervous system. *Brain*, **131**, 1171–96.

Jones AK, Cunningham VJ, Ha-Kawa S, Fujiwara T, Luthra SK, Silva S et al. (1994). Changes in central opioid receptor binding in relation to inflammation and pain in patients with rheumatoid arthritis. *British Journal of Rheumatology*, **33**, 909–16.

Jones AK, Kitchen ND, Watabe H, Cunningham VJ, Jones T, Luthra SK et al. (1999). Measurement of changes in opioid receptor binding in vivo during trigeminal neuralgic pain using [11C] diprenorphine and positron emission tomography. *Journal of Cerebral Blood Flow & Metabolism*, **19**, 803–8.

Jones AKP, Kulkarni B, and Derbyshire SWG (2003). Pain mechanisms and their disorders: imaging in clinical neuroscience. *British Medical Bulletin*, **65**, 83–93.

Jones AK, Qi LY, Fujirawa T, Luthra SK, Ashburner J, Bloomfield P et al. (1991). *In vivo* distribution of opioid receptors in man in relation to the cortical projections of the medial and lateral pain systems measured with positron emission tomography. *Neuroscience Letters*, **126**, 25–8.

Jones AK, Watabe H, Cunningham VJ, and Jones T (2004). Cerebral decreases in opioid receptor binding in patients with central neuropathic pain measured by [11C]diprenorphine binding and PET. *European Journal of Pain*, **8**, 479–85.

Maarrawi J, Peyron R, Mertens P, Costes N, Magnin M, Sindou M et al. (2007). Differential brain opioid receptor availability in central and peripheral neuropathic pain. *Pain*, **127**, 183–94.

Mueller C, Klega A, Buchholz HG, Rolke R, Magerl W, Schirrmacher R et al. (2010). Basal opioid receptor binding is associated with differences in sensory perception in healthy human subjects: a [18F]diprenorphine PET study. *NeuroImage*, **49**, 731–7.

Petrovic P, Kalso E, Petersson KM, and Ingvar M (2002). Placebo and opioid analgesia–imaging a shared neuronal network. *Science*, **295**, 1737–40.

Smith YR, Stohler CS, Nichols TE, Bueller JA, Koeppe RA, and Zubieta JK (2006). Pronociceptive and antinociceptive effects of estradiol through endogenous opioid neurotransmission in women. *Journal of Neuroscience*, **26**, 5777–85.

Sprenger T, Valet M, Boecker H, Henriksen G, Spilker ME, Willoch F et al. (2006). Opioidergic activation in the medial pain system after heat pain. *Pain*, **122**, 63–7.

Turner R and Jones T (2003). Techniques for imaging neuroscience. *British Medical Bulletin*, **65**, 3–20.

Willoch F, Schindler F, Wester HJ, Empl M, Straube A, Schwaiger M et al. (2004). Central post-stroke pain and reduced opioid receptor binding within pain processing circuitries: a [11C] diprenorphine PET study. *Pain*, **108**, 213–20.

Zubieta JK, Bueller JA, Jackson LR, Scott DJ, Xu Y, Koeppe RA et al. (2005). Placebo effects mediated by endogenous opioid activity on mu-opioid receptors. *Journal of Neuroscience*, **25**, 7754–62.

Zubieta JK, Dannals RF, and Frost JJ (1999). Gender and age influences on human brain mu-opioid receptor binding measured by PET. *American Journal of Psychiatry*, **156**, 842–8.

Zubieta JK, Heitzeg MM, Smith YR, Bueller JA, Xu K, Xu Y et al. (2003). COMT val158met genotype affects mu-opioid neurotransmitter responses to a pain stressor. *Science*, **299**, 1240–3.

Zubieta JK, Smith YR, Bueller JA, Xu Y, Kilbourn MR, Jewett DM et al. (2001). Regional mu opioid receptor regulation of sensory and affective dimensions of pain. *Science*, **293**, 311–15.

Chapter 4

Opioid pharmacogenomics

Key points

- Pharmacogenomic phenotypes account for some of the inter-individual variations in opioid response.
- This is best exemplified by variations in the metabolic pathways for codeine and tramadol.
- There are common functional variants in opiate receptors, but, as yet, the clinical significance of these polymorphisms is uncertain.

4.1 Introduction

The burgeoning field of pharmacogenomics holds the promise to personalize therapeutics on the basis of metabolic, pharmacodynamic, and a myriad of interacting genetic phenotypes that are the product of variations in the individual's genome. This promise is now being realized in some therapeutic areas such as using tumour pharmacogenomics to direct rational cancer treatment. The opiate receptors have attracted considerable attention from the earliest days of pharmacogenomics, as explanations were sought for the known variable responses of individuals to opiates in terms of both efficacy and side effects. These studies were given additional impetus by the knowledge that the opiate receptors come from single genes, with identified genetic variants that altered their function. Additionally, polymorphisms at a number of other gene locations, including in metabolic pathways, have been shown to exert influences (sometimes dramatic) on a number of opioids, including codeine and tramadol. The bulk of the studies, to date, have used hypothesis-driven approaches to explore the impact of polymorphisms in genes of known significance.

4.1.1 Opiate receptor polymorphisms

Gene knock-out of the μ-OR (OPRM1) in mice completely removes the analgesic action of systemically administered opiates, along with many of the significant side effects, identifying this locus as a key determinate of opioid analgesic actions. Much work has, therefore, focused on the presence of single nucleotide polymorphisms (SNPs) in this locus (of which over 100 are known, albeit mostly rare in the population). There are pedigrees with completely dysfunctional μ-OR, but these appear to be rare in the population, and their pain phenotype is not well characterized. A common μ-OR polymorphism (A118G, present in >10% of Caucasians) has been extensively investigated and is associated with 2–3-fold decrease in sensitivity to opiates, both in terms of analgesic efficacy and side effects such as respiratory depression, in volunteer studies. However, in clinical practice, this apparent effect has not been discriminated in a meta-analysis of patient studies where no clear difference was found in either opiate dosing, pain scores, or side effect profile. Although this is only one variant (with a moderate phenotype), this analysis has perhaps diminished the likelihood that prior pharmacogenetic screening for μ-OR SNPs will usefully inform prescribing practice because of the multifactorial influences on pain perception.

4.1.2 Polymorphisms in metabolic pathways

The actions of several opiates are dependent upon metabolic pathways, either because they are pro-drugs (like codeine, which is converted to morphine) or their activity depends on the presence of active metabolites (e.g. tramadol). In both these cases, their conversion is catalysed by a particular isoform (CYP2D6) of the P450 super-family of phase I metabolic enzymes. The CYP2D6 gene has both poor and ultrafast metabolizer (PM and UM, respectively) phenotypes, each of which occurs with a frequency of around 7% in the Caucasian population. Patients with a PM phenotype will obtain little analgesic benefit from codeine, whereas the UM gene leads to a risk of toxic levels of morphine. These variations account for part (but not all) of the inter-individual variation seen in response to codeine (leading to a high NNT) and have also led to a specific warning about the use of codeine in breastfeeding mothers because of the risk of infant poisoning if the mother has the UM genotype. This could make a rationale for genotyping before codeine prescription, but pragmatic clinical practice would probably avoid codeine prescribing altogether because of its inherent variability of response.

The situation with tramadol is less black and white, as, although its O-desmethyltramadol metabolite is a potent μ-OR agonist and its levels are dependent upon the CYP2D6 phenotype, the drug is active both at μ-OR in its own right and also at monoamine re-uptake sites. Notably however, studies have shown that variation in the analgesic response to tramadol in post-operative patients is related to the CYP2D6 genotype.

The elimination of several opiates depends on hepatic metabolism. An example is fentanyl, which is dependent upon CYP3A4 that also has PM and UM phenotypes. Clinical studies in Asian populations have shown a relationship between the dose requirement and genotype. Morphine also undergoes glucuronidation by phase II metabolic enzymes to either active morphine-6-glucuronide or to the inactive morphine-3-glucuronide. These enzymes are known to have functional polymorphisms, but, as yet, a clinically relevant phenotype has not been identified.

4.1.3 Interaction with synergistic pathways

It is appreciated from animal studies that there are bidirectional interactions between opioid analgesics and endogenous monaminergic neural systems, including norepinephrine and 5-HT, whereby depletion of monoamines reduces the analgesic efficacy of opiates. On this basis, considerable attention has focused on the relationship between SNPs in re-uptake (SERT and NET) and metabolic pathways (MAO and COMT) for the monoamines, and their influence on responses to opiates. To date, there have been relatively few positive findings from these studies, with the exception of COMT.

COMT

Catechol-o-methyl transferase is one of the main metabolic enzymes for norepinephrine and dopamine and shows common phenotype variation in its activity. An SNP that reduces its activity (increasing monoamine levels) has been linked with both increased pain perception to a standardized stimulus and an increase in the sensitivity to morphine (by more than 50%). Although the change in pain responsiveness has been challenged in patient populations, it appears that the link to opiate sensitivity (exogenous and endogenous) is reproducible if moderate in magnitude. Furthermore, there is evidence from PET imaging studies that these changes correlate with differences in the degree of activation of the endogenous opioid system.

4.2 **Clinical relevance**

As yet, the evidence threshold has not been crossed to mandate the routine introduction of genotyping to direct opioid therapy; yet, sufficient data have accumulated to indicate that there will be phenotypes that account for a proportion of the large variability both in pain responses to similar insults and the sensitivity to opioid benefits and side effect. The list of hypothesized 'pain genes' for investigation becomes wider, with recognition of new therapeutic targets for intervention. However, based on pioneering animal studies that identified genetic loci associated with large strain variations in pain and analgesic sensitivity, there is a sound rationale for genome-wide association studies in man to identify equivalent genetic fingerprints. It seems likely that the results of such studies will (once the cost-benefit debate has been fought) significantly alter our current, largely empirical opioid prescribing practice for individuals.

Key Reading

Lotsch J and Geisslinger G (2006). Relevance of frequent mu-opioid receptor polymorphisms for opioid activity in healthy volunteers. *Pharmacogenomics Journal*, **6**, 200–10.

Lotsch J and Geisslinger G (2011). Pharmacogenetics of new analgesics. *British Journal of Pharmacology*, **163**, 447–60.

Matthes HW, Maldonado R, Simonin F, Valverde O, Slowe S, Kitchen I et al. (1996). Loss of morphine-induced analgesia, reward effect and withdrawal symptoms in mice lacking the mu-opioid-receptor gene. *Nature*, **383**, 819–23.

Mogil JS (2009). Are we getting anywhere in human pain genetics? Pain, **146**, 231–2.

Muralidharan A and Smith MT (2011). Pain, analgesia and genetics. *Journal of Pharmacy and Pharmacology*, **63**, 1387–400.

Walter C and Lotsch J (2009). Meta-analysis of the relevance of the OPRM1 118A>G genetic variant for pain treatment. *Pain*, **146**, 270–5.

Zubieta JK, Heitzeg MM, Smith YR, Bueller JA, Xu K, Xu Y et al. (2003). COMT val158met genotype affects mu-opioid neurotransmitter responses to a pain stressor. *Science*, **299**, 1240–3.

Chapter 5

Opioid prescribing trends: an international perspective

The relaxation of restrictive opioid laws in the US towards the end of the last century, a recognition of the disabling burden of chronic pain, and the emergence of trial data, albeit short-term, suggesting that opioids have a role in the management of long-term pain have resulted in a climate of increasing willingness to prescribe opioids. There has been a marked and progressive rise in the prescription of opioid drugs in both the UK and the US over the last decade.

Raw prescribing data do not answer all the questions about who is prescribing which drugs, in what doses and for which indication. Nonetheless, the per capita consumption of therapeutic opioids in the US increased by 400% in the decade 1997–2007, with the increases for oxycodone and methadone being over 800% and nearly 1300%, respectively. Similar rises occurred in the UK, with the per capita consumption increasing by nearly 300% in the same period and an overall doubling of prescription opioid items dispensed. In Australia, opioid prescriptions have increased threefold in this period, with a doubling of per capita opioid consumption. Global data are comparable, with the sharpest rises occurring in developed nations. Although an increase in opioid prescribing might be seen as a surrogate marker of the imperative to better recognize and manage persistent pain, the promise of reducing the burden of persistent pain has not been fulfilled. This is not surprising, given the more recent conclusions from the published literature on opioid efficacy, which suggest that the effectiveness of prescribing opioids in the long term may be limited, evidence of the drugs bringing about improvement in quality of life is lacking, and persistent pain remains as refractory to this potent group of drugs as it does to other medication classes and therapeutic interventions. Emerging data suggest that the increasing use of opioids for persistent pain imposes an additional set of harm for patients with pain, and for society. Risks of fractures, overdose, and emergency department visits increase with increasing dose of opioids, and higher doses are more frequently prescribed to individuals who are at more risk of running into problems: the so-called adverse selection.

Data from the US, Australia, and elsewhere clearly demonstrate increase in prescription drug misuse (described by the US Centre for Disease Control as an epidemic) and additional risk of overdose and death, in parallel with the rise in prescription of opioids, and identification and management of patients who may misuse or divert opioid drugs has been an intense focus of research. Data from the UK indicate that addiction to prescribed and over-the-counter analgesic medication does occur, but to a much lesser extent, and the rate of rise of the problem has, to date, been modest. Review of the most recent data from Office of National Statistics on drug-related deaths shows a rise in deaths related to methadone (used in the UK almost exclusively as opioid substitution therapy) from 2006 to 2010, with no rise in morphine-related deaths, a plateauing of deaths relating to codeine, but a continued steady increase in tramadol deaths. At the time of writing, concern from groups representing patients addicted to medicines and from professionals treating pain and addiction, particularly in the context of the transatlantic experience of opioid misuse, has prompted a coordinated governmental appraisal of the problem and the development of a strategy to minimize further individual and societal harm in relation to opioid medications.

Key Reading

Boudreau D, Von Korff M, Rutter CM, Saunders K, Ray GT, Sullivan MD et al. (2009). Trends in long-term opioid therapy for chronic non-cancer pain. *Pharmacoepidemiology and Drug Safety*, **18**, 1166–75.

Caudill-Slosberg MA, Schwartz LM, and Woloshin S (2004). Office visits and analgesic prescriptions for musculoskeletal pain in US: 1980 versus 2000. *Pain*, **109**, 514–19.

Dunn KM, Saunders KW, Rutter CM, Banta-Green CJ, Merrill JO, Sullivan MD et al. (2010). Opioid prescriptions for chronic pain and overdose. *Annals of Internal Medicine*, **152**, 85–92.*

Manchikanti L and Singh A (2008). Therapeutic opioids: a ten-year perspective on the complexities and complications of the escalating use, abuse, and non-medical use of opioids. *Pain Physician*, **11**, S63–88.

National Treatment Agency for Substance Misuse (2011). Addiction to medicine. Available from: http://www.nta.nhs.uk/uploads/addictiontomedicinesmay2011a.pdf [Accessed November 26, 2012].

NHS Information Centre (n.d.). Prescriptions. Available from: www.ic.nhs.uk/statistics-and-data-collections/primary-care/prescriptions [Accessed March 18, 2012].

Office for National Statistics (2010). Deaths related to drug poisoning in England and Wales, 2010. Available from: http://www.ons.gov.uk/ons/rel/subnational-health3/deaths-related-to-drug-poisoning/2010/stb-deaths-related-to-drug-poisoning-2010.html [Accessed November 26, 2012].

Substance Abuse and Mental Health Services Administration (2009). Results from the 2008 National Survey on Drug Use and Health: National Findings (Office of Applied Studies, NSDUH Series H-36, DHHS Publication No. SMA 09-4434). Rockville, MD. Available from: http://www.oas.samhsa.gov [Accessed November 26, 2012].

Sullivan MD, Edlund MJ, Fan MY, Devries A, Brennan Braden J, and Martin BC (2008). Trends in use of opioids for non-cancer pain conditions 2000–2005 in commercial and Medicaid insurance plans: The TROUP study. *Pain*, **138**, 440–9.

Sullivan MD (2011). Limiting the potential harms of high-dose opioid therapy. *Archives of Internal Medicine*, **171**, 691–2.

Von Korff M and Deyo R (2004). Potent opioids for chronic musculoskeletal pain: flying blind? *Pain*, **109**, 207–9.

---

* Important paper which shows that potentially lethal harms of opioid therapy may be dose-related.

Chapter 6

Current good practice in pain medicine

Key points

- Pain is a complex sensory and emotional experience upon which there are numerous influences.
- Pain is related to dysfunction physically, socially, emotionally, and vocationally.
- Techniques for the management of acute pain have poor applicability to the management of persisting symptoms.
- Assessment of pain should include evaluation of patients' beliefs about their symptoms, and an exploration of the impact of symptoms on the patient's life.
- Trust between patient and therapist underpins successful pain management.

6.1 Experiencing pain

Pain is a complex sensory and emotional experience, and its determinants are not only biological processes which may, to varying degrees, result in initiation and transmission of injury signals in pain processing pathways but also to numerous other modulating influences, including previous experience, expectation, and social context. In addition, the attitudes and beliefs of those with whom the individual with pain comes into contact will shape the experience of pain and the response to therapy. The integrated cerebral circuitry by which these influences modify the perceptual experience of pain and its consequences, such as anxiety and fear, is being revealed by neuroimaging techniques such as positron emission tomography (PET) and functional magnetic resonance imaging (fMRI). These techniques are demonstrating the profound structural and functional changes that occur in the central nervous system as the result of, or as antecedents to, chronic pain. Any treatment, be it physical, pharmacological, or psychological, must be continually re-evaluated within this rapidly evolving context and in the light of the contemporary evidence base.

6.1.1 Pain and function

As complex as the neurobiological correlates of pain perception are the many ways in which pain can affect the individual. For many, persistent pain can infiltrate all aspects of physical, social, emotional, and vocational function, and it can escape the physical confines of the immediate sufferer and come to affect the lives of his or her family and carers. It is tempting to regard dysfunction in these various domains solely as a consequence of the presence of chronic pain. If this were so, the only goal of therapy would be to reduce the intensity of pain. Experience has shown not only that this is often difficult but also that the assumption that, in emotional, social, or vocational domains, dysfunction has no causal influence on how we perceive pain leads to therapeutic disappointment for both the patient and the professional.

6.1.2 Managing acute and chronic pain

The management of acute pain focuses on identifying the potential source of tissue damage and employing rational strategies to modify nociceptive input whilst healing occurs. In contrast, chronic pain management strategies recognize that modifying the perception of pain has to go hand-in-hand with support for the patient in making improvements to his or her levels of physical and psychological function, and quality of life. When assessing patients with chronic pain, it is important to remember that they are likely to have had many previous contacts with sources of help for their symptoms. These may have been intensely frustrating, and perhaps counterproductive, interactions for both the professional, who feels impotent in the face of complaints that fail to fit the usual symptom-diagnosis-treatment model, and the patient whose symptoms persist unabated.

By its nature, pain is an intensely personal experience and is remarkably difficult to describe. This can lead patients to feel isolated not only from health professionals but also from friends and relatives.

As Virginia Woolf said in her essay 'On being ill',

> English, which can express the thoughts of Hamlet and the tragedy of Lear has no words for the … headache … The merest schoolgirl when she falls in love has Shakespeare or Keats to speak her mind for her, but let a sufferer try to describe a pain in his head to a doctor and language at once runs dry.

Woolf was writing of the headache, a pain everyone has experienced. How much more relevant it is to the pain of a phantom limb or that following a stroke. This poverty of language can be a significant barrier within therapeutic relationships, and disbelief of those with pain is not uncommon. Developing a relationship of mutual trust between the patient and the therapist is an important first step in successful management.

6.1.3 Assessment of the patient with pain

Initial assessment of the patient should include not only biomedical evaluation of past or current potentially injurious pathology but also social, cultural, and emotional contributors to, and consequences of, pain. It is important to explore the patients' understanding of their pain, and symptoms should be explained to them from an appropriate and understandable perspective. Concurrent mood and anxiety disorders should be identified, as they may, if left untreated, preclude successful pain management. Results of clinical investigations, including radiological imaging techniques, should be interpreted with caution. X-rays and scans illuminate only part of the problem and, because of the high prevalence of 'abnormal' structural findings in the asymptomatic population, they can act as a distraction when trying to formulate a pain management plan.

For the non-specialist in pain management, careful evaluation of the patient, including an assessment of the effects that pain has had on the patient's life, is a good starting point for management. More complex cases will ideally be assessed and treated by a multidisciplinary team, including physical therapists, pain psychologists, and specialists in pain medicine. Such teams can deliver a range of physical, pharmacological, and behavioural interventions, often in parallel.

6.2 The role of opioids in pain management

Expectations regarding what opioid medications can achieve in the management of persistent pain need to be realistically rooted, and data to support effectiveness when opioids are prescribed in the long term are lacking. In addition to their role in mediating analgesia, opioid drugs and endogenous opioid peptides have an impact on, and play a role in, numerous and diverse biological and behavioural processes, including affective state, motivation, arousal and sleep, endocrine, gastric and hepatic function, and immune processes. They have well-recognized effects on the respiratory, cardiovascular, and nervous systems, including aspects of learning and memory. Opioids might be expected to benefit many aspects and consequences of the pain experience, but, somewhat surprisingly, the primary goal of opioid therapy remains a reduction in pain intensity. Whilst most contemporary studies regarding the efficacy of analgesics recognize that improvement in quality of life is an additional, important outcome measure, the use of opioids to improve, for example, mood, sleep, and anxiety, is cautioned against if the primary goal of analgesia is not achieved.

6.2.1 Weak and strong opioids

Opioids are traditionally divided into 'weak' and 'strong'. This is based on the relative potencies of the drugs but is ultimately an unhelpful distinction, as opioids are used over very wide dose ranges, and 'weak' opioids are often used far in excess of the published maximum dose. Furthermore, all the opioids exert the majority of their effects via the ORs (in particular, the μ-OR), whether or not they are classed as weak or strong. They show dose-dependent pharmacodynamics, which further underlines the arbitrary nature of the division. Most of the published trial data presented in this text relate to the use of 'strong' opioid preparations.

Table 6.1 Examples of non-injectable opioids available in the UK	
Strong opioids	
Approved name (some proprietary names)	Formulations available
Buprenorphine	Sublingual, transdermal
Dipipanone	Oral
Fentanyl	Transdermal, transmucosal, oral
Hydromorphone	Oral
Methadone	Oral
Morphine	Oral
Oxycodone	Oral

Table 6.1 *(Contd.)*	
Strong opioids	
Approved name (some proprietary names)	Formulations available
Pentazocine	Oral
Pethidine	Oral
Tapentadol	Oral
Tramadol	Oral
Weak opioids	
Codeine	Oral
Dextropropoxyphene	Oral
Dihydrocodeine	Oral
Meptazinol	Oral

Oral formulations may be immediate or modified release.

Reproduced with permission from the British Pain Society (2010). Recommendations for the appropriate use of opioids in persistent non-cancer pain. Available from: http://www.britishpainsociety.org/book_opioid_main.pdf [Accessed September 2012].

Some of the opioids are presented with paracetamol as compound analgesic preparations, e.g. co-codamol, Kapake®, Solpadol®, Tylex®, co-dydramol, Remedeine®, and co-proxamol. Some opioids are presented with anti-emetics as compound preparations, e.g. Diconal® (dipipanone and cyclizine). See BNF for more details.

Table 6.1 lists examples of non-injectable opioids, currently available in the UK. For clarity, we have maintained the customary division into weak and strong opioids.

Key Reading

Carr DB, Morris DB, and Loeser JD (eds.) (2005). *Narrative, pain, and suffering*. IASP Press, Seattle.

Melzack R and Wall P (1996). *The challenge of pain*. 2nd edn. Penguin, London.

Morris DB (1993). *The culture of pain*. University of California Press, Berkeley.

Wall P (2000). *Pain: the science of suffering*. Phoenix, London.

Chapter 7

Benefits and adverse effects of opioids

Key points

- Opioids may help some people with long-term pain and may also have a beneficial effect on sleep and mood.
- There is weak evidence only that opioid use can improve physical function.
- Psychomotor function may not be degraded by chronic opioid treatment.
- The law on driving whilst taking prescribed opioids varies between countries.
- Opioids are associated with a wide range of adverse effects that need to be weighed against any benefits to judge the overall effectiveness of treatment.

7.1 Introduction

One of the most potent areas of controversy surrounding opioid prescribing involves the setting of appropriate treatment aims. The primary treatment goal of acute pain and cancer pain is a reduction in pain intensity. In chronic non-malignant pain, however, treatment aims also include improvements in sleep and mood, enhanced physical and social function, and psychological well-being. Whether an improvement in one or more of these domains, in the absence of a reduction in pain intensity, should constitute a treatment success is unclear. What is less controversial is that opioids are best used as part of an integrated rehabilitation programme, aimed at improving physical, emotional, and social function, not simply to provide pain relief.

7.2 Benefits of opioids

Analgesia is the primary outcome measure when judging the effectiveness of opioid treatment. In a systematic review of opioid effectiveness, the average (mean) pain relief with opioids was 30% in both neuropathic and nociceptive pain. All the trials included in the review used validated measures of pain intensity, and this degree of pain relief reached the threshold of what is usually thought to be clinically significant analgesia. However, these interpretations may be favourable, and more critical review, particularly in relation to how data from trial non-completers may be managed, suggests that opioids may help fewer patients than indicated by current systematic reviews. The effects of opioids on other pain-related sensations, such as static or dynamic allodynia, are reviewed in the section on neuropathic pain.

Secondary outcome measures, such as impact on sleep, mood, quality of life, and physical functioning, are also addressed by a number of randomized clinical trials. These data are often difficult to interpret, and the methodology is sometimes difficult to determine from the published material. The validity of secondary outcome measures is further compromised by the short duration of most of the trials where the blinded phases last, at most, 2 months, and the open-label phases 2 years. However, there is consistent evidence that opioid use may result in improved self-reported quality of sleep, particularly in subjects who derive analgesic benefit from opioids.

Measures of depression tend to remain unchanged during opioid treatment. Mood has been specifically addressed in only two randomized controlled trials. Both of these trials reported a significant improvement in mood that was dependent on analgesic efficacy.

Most high-quality trials of opioids have reported the effects of oral opioid therapy on various aspects of quality of life, but only three have used a validated measure, two trials using the SF-36 and one trial the Sickness Impact Profile. Only one of these three trials has reported a significant improvement in a number of the quality-of-life domains of the SF-36.

There is evidence from intravenous testing of opioids that opioids can improve physical function. One study of subjects with chronic low back pain reported increased back strength and endurance following intravenous fentanyl, but the majority of studies using longer-term oral dosing with opioids have failed to show any beneficial effect of opioids on self-reported levels of overall ability or pain-related interference in daily activities, walking ability, pain disability index, physical function, or general activity. Two studies have shown that disability scores are reduced during treatment with oxycodone compared to placebo, and one study has demonstrated that improvement in pain-related disability is closely related to analgesic effect.

Current evidence does not suggest consistent degradation of psychomotor skills with opioid use (see Undesirable effects of opioids on driving). Conversely, the presence of cancer pain is known to reduce psychomotor performance, so one could hypothesize that adequate treatment of chronic non-cancer pain with opioids could result in an improvement in psychomotor function. This is yet to be convincingly demonstrated experimentally.

There are some data from large cross-sectional studies that give us more insight into the possible long-term results of opioid treatment on the domains mentioned in this section. In one such study, opioid use was associated with poorer self-rated health, poorer quality of life in all domains of SF-36, higher health care consumption, and unemployment, even when the data were controlled for pain intensity. Although these are cross-sectional data, and longitudinal data are still required, this study throws doubt on the ability of chronic opioid therapy to effect significant improvements on long-term physical, psychological, and socio-economic function.

7.3 **Undesirable effects of opioids**

When judging the appropriateness of any intervention, the benefits conferred as a result of treatment have to be weighed against effects that are detrimental to the patient's physical or psychological well-being. This applies particularly to treatment with opioids, which are a class of drugs that have a wide range of undesirable effects and which may confer marginal benefits only. Adverse events are common during treatment with strong opioids. A systematic review of placebo-controlled trials showed that 80% of patients treated with opioids experienced at least one adverse effect, compared with 56% of patients receiving placebo. Another way to present these data is to say that the number needed to harm is 4.2, i.e. if four patients are treated with opioids, one more will experience an undesirable effect than if they were treated with placebo. Another systematic review (which included non-placebo-controlled trials) demonstrated that around 50% of patients experienced at least one adverse effect, which was of sufficient severity to cause 22% of patients to withdraw from their respective trials. Most of the data on adverse effects come from studies of short duration, and, in many of these trials, the dose was not titrated against beneficial and adverse effects but was administered in accordance with a strict protocol. This limits the applicability of the data to everyday clinical care. There is little evidence that any particular opioid is less likely to cause clinically significant adverse effects than any other, and studies purporting to support that claim often use non-equianalgesic doses.

7.3.1 Gastrointestinal adverse effects

Constipation and nausea are the most common adverse events associated with opioid use, their frequency being related to the intensity of the pain treated and, by inference, the opioid dose used. Constipation affects approximately 40% of patients taking opioids for chronic pain and is both the most common side effect, and one of the most difficult to treat. Some authorities have claimed that transdermal fentanyl is less likely to cause constipation than oral morphine, but the methodology of the trials upon which that claim rests has been questioned. Unlike other adverse effects, constipation tends not to settle with prolonged opioid use and, in the setting of chronic pain, may often be exacerbated by a lack of physical activity. Additionally, the patient may be receiving other medications that are constipating such as the tricyclic antidepressants. It is prudent, therefore, to prescribe prophylactic aperients when starting opioids, but there is little guidance in the scientific literature to aid the choice of laxative. A common sense approach is to use both a stool softener along with a bowel stimulant. An alternative strategy has been developed, using the administration of naloxone via the gastrointestinal tract to block the gut μ-OR while leaving the central opiate analgesic effects unchanged. While this is a potentially interesting approach, as yet, the evidence base supporting its clinical deployment is limited (see Chapter 2).

Clinical experience has demonstrated that constipation tends to be a persistent problem during the course of treatment, and patients may need to take laxatives until they stop taking opioids. Nausea, by contrast, tends to settle with time but is still experienced by around 30% of patients. Multiple mechanisms may be involved: opioid-induced emetogenesis, including the activation of the chemoreceptor trigger zone (CTZ), gastric stasis, and effects on the vestibular system. Resistant nausea may, therefore, require multimodal treatment. The dopamine antagonist metoclopramide may be useful as a first-line treatment. It exerts its anti-emetic effect by blocking central D2 receptors, leading to an increased threshold for vomiting in the CTZ, and by peripheral D2 receptor blockade that induces gastric peristalsis and increases gastrointestinal motility. The serotonin antagonists (e.g. ondansetron) may also be useful, as they have a superior safety profile and may be better tolerated than the dopamine antagonists. Theoretically, they may reduce the analgesic efficacy of tramadol, which exerts a portion of its effects via the 5-HT system, but this is yet to be proven in human studies. It is the authors' practice to prescribe prophylactic anti-emetics when starting opioid treatment, but long-term anti-emetics are rarely necessary. Vomiting is relatively uncommon, experienced by only one in ten patients but, nevertheless, is a distressing side effect that can result in cessation of treatment.

7.3.2 **Effects on psychomotor function, cognitive function, and the ability to drive**

As the use of opioid medication to treat chronic non-cancer pain has become more widely accepted, it has become more important to be able to give evidence-based advice to patients regarding their ability to drive. Discussion about the effects of pain and medication on driving are an important part of consent to treatment. The effects of each medication vary between individuals, and the impact on driving will also be affected by pain and associated disability, fatigue and sleeplessness, and other medications that the patient is taking. The Driver and Vehicle Licensing Agency (DVLA) advises that a patient should not drive if their ability to do so is impaired. A patient has a responsibility to consider their fitness on each occasion they wish to drive. DVLA's current medical standards of fitness to drive does not give guidance on pain and analgesia (other than in relation to recovery from surgery).

When discussing implications of opioid therapy for driving, it is important to make clear that impairment is most likely at initiation of pain medication therapy and at times of dose adjustment, and that the balance of benefits and harms of treatments must be considered in each case. Patients should be made aware that they may only achieve useful pain relief at medication doses that make them unfit to drive. Health care professionals must ensure that patients understand the rationale behind driving laws, and that concerns regarding fitness to drive relate to their safety and that of others.

It is important that patients with pain, who wish to take analgesic medication, comply with the requirements of their motor vehicle insurer in relation to disclosure of information regarding physical impairment and medication.

Driving whilst taking illicit or prescribed opioids is specifically outlawed in many countries, regardless of whether an individual's driving performance is affected. There are some exceptions to this amongst European Union countries. These include France where the law protects patients taking prescribed drugs from prosecution, Austria where drug taking has to be accompanied by an obvious reduction in driving performance to violate the law, and Germany where the situation is similar. In the UK, opioid use is only an absolute bar to holding a driving licence when it constitutes misuse or dependency, although, at the time of writing, UK drug driving laws are under review.

This position is broadly in harmony with the scientific evidence base. Early studies, looking at cognitive and psychomotor function in opioid-naive subjects given a single-dose challenge with an opioid, demonstrated a degradation in motor coordination, brief and sustained attention, and short-term memory. This is the basis of the advice that patients refrain from driving during upwards opioid dose titration. When one looks to the evidence base regarding stable opioid treatment, it consistently demonstrates that stable doses do not impair psychomotor abilities related to driving and, furthermore, that opioid users have no greater incidence of motor vehicle accidents than the general population. In studies using driving simulators, again the evidence tells us that opioids do not significantly impair driving skills. The evidence relating to cognitive function is less clear, with some studies showing that opioid users have significantly reduced cognitive function (including impairment of memory), whilst others show little difference. There is strong evidence, however, that unrelieved pain reduces both psychomotor and cognitive ability, so the reduction in cognitive function that may occur as a result of opioid use has to be seen in this context. The use of other sedative drugs, such as alcohol or benzodiazepines, at the same time as opioids significantly impairs psychomotor abilities and is, therefore an absolute contraindication to driving. Although a recent systematic review concludes that high-quality evidence suggests that opioids used for long periods do not impair cognitive function, it points out that the analysis of studies, which may be methodologically somewhat flawed, suggests a degree of uncertainty regarding firm conclusions in relation to cognitive effects.

7.3.3 Opioid-induced myoclonus

A number of movement abnormalities are associated in a dose-related manner with the use of opioids. The frequency of occurrence is variably reported. Myoclonus describes an involuntary and uncontrollable jerking of various muscle groups, usually in the limbs. The neuropharmacology is not well defined. One hypothesis is that it is related to the accumulation of neuroexcitatory metabolites, e.g. morphine-3-glucuronide, and, in particular, a high M3G/M6G ratio is thought to be unfavourable. Accumulation of morphine metabolites in those with impaired renal function can be associated with generalized myoclonus, which can improve when the patient is switched to an alternative opioid. The observation that the phenomenon seems to be more prominent in those receiving oral versus parenteral morphine has been linked to hepatic metabolism.

Other mechanisms postulated include an antagonist effect of opioids on inhibitory peptides in the spinal cord, such as GABA and glycine, resulting in depolarization of spinal neurones. Myoclonus may also relate to central serotonergic and dopaminergic effects of opioids. The problem is likely to be increased in individuals with pre-existing neurologic disorder and in those receiving other drugs, such as haloperidol or prochlorperazine, that have anti-dopaminergic properties.

Myoclonus may be treated by reducing opioid dose or by opioid switching. Muscle relaxants, such as benzodiazepines, baclofen, or dantrolene, have also been reported as usefully attenuating the symptom.

7.3.4 Endocrine effects of opioids

Under physiological conditions, the endogenous opioid system and the endocrine system are closely interlinked. Endogenous opioids, such as beta-endorphin, are involved in the regulation of gonadotrophin-releasing hormone (GnRH) and adrenocorticotrophic hormone. It is, therefore, not surprising that exogenous opioids can adversely affect endocrine function.

Hypothalamic-pituitary-gonadal axis

Of all the hypothalamic endocrine functions, the effect of opioids on the hypothalamic-pituitary-gonadal axis is the most profound. The hypothalamus secretes GnRH that flows into the pituitary in the hypophyseal portal circulation. In the anterior pituitary, GnRH stimulates follicle-stimulating hormone (FSH) and luteinizing hormone (LH).

Primary hypogonadism is the result of gonadal failure. Secondary hypogonadism is the result of failure of the hypothalamic-pituitary-gonadal axis at the hypothalamic or pituitary levels; chronic opioid use is a cause of secondary hypogonadism. Both endogenous and exogenous opioids reduce the normal pulsatile nature of GnRH release from the hypothalamus, resulting in a fall in LH and FSH secretion from the pituitary. In the male, this leads to a reduction in testosterone release from the testes and, in the female, a reduction in progesterone and oestrogen release from the ovaries. In the male, this can lead to erectile dysfunction, loss of libido, and a reduction in muscle mass, and, in the female, amenorrhoea, a reduction in breast size, and menopausal symptoms. In both sexes, infertility, mood disturbance, hyperglycaemia, hypercholesterolaemia, gynaeco-mastia, galactorrhoea, fatigue, osteoporosis, and night sweats may occur.

Other endocrine effects
The effect of opioid treatment on growth hormone is complex and poorly under-stood. Acute administration of opioids increases the production of growth hormone, but, in one study of patients on long-term intrathecal opioid therapy, 15% of patients exhibited low growth hormone levels. A similar proportion of patients demonstrated hypocortisolism, and there have been rare occurrences of Addisonian crises in patients on high-dose opioid therapy. Occasionally, opioid administration can result in increased prolactin release from the anterior pituitary, although the clinical significance of this is doubtful. Long-term opioid therapy can increase tonic sympathetic activity, and patients on such therapy need to be monitored for hypertension. Lastly, it is known that the endogenous opioid system is involved in food-related reward mechanisms, and chronic opioid therapy is associated with weight gain and poor blood sugar regulation. This may be via mechanisms separate from the hyperglycaemia seen as part of an opioid-induced hypogonadal syndrome.

Management
Opioid-induced endocrine effects, in particular, opioid-induced hypogonadism, are now so well recognized that it is mandatory to include a discussion of these effects with patients prior to a trial of long-term opioid therapy. Some authorities recommend measuring thyroid function, sex hormone levels, and bone density in patients prior to starting opioid treatment, and repeating hormone assays 6-monthly thereafter. If endo-crine dysfunction is suspected, then consideration should be given to stopping opioid treatment to see if symptoms resolve. If this is not possible, then hormone replace-ment should be undertaken under shared care with an endocrinologist.

7.3.5 **Immune modulation**

It is known that opioids are immunomodulatory, but the mechanisms of this phenom-enon are complex and the clinical implications unclear. Opioids can affect antibody production, natural killer (NK) lymphocytic activity, cytokine expression, and phago-cyte activity. Many of these effects have been studied in intravenous drug users, some of whom have HIV infection, and methadone has been described as a co-factor in the development of AIDS. In addition, animal studies have demonstrated increased cancer spread in animals treated with some opioids.

As might be expected, morphine is the opioid for which the immunomodulatory effect has been most closely studied. It is thought that morphine has both direct and indirect effects on the immune response. It binds to μ-receptors on a range of immune cells, including T lymphocytes, B lymphocytes, NK lymphocytes, monocytes, and mac-rophages. Opioids also activate the hypothalamic-pituitary-adrenal axis and the sympa-thetic nervous system, resulting in the release of glucocorticoids and norepinephrine, both of which adversely affect leucocyte function.

From animal studies, we know that some opioids have greater effects on immune function than others. Opioids fall into two groups: those that have significant immuno-suppressive actions (codeine, methadone, morphine, fentanyl), and those that cause less immunosuppression (buprenorphine, hydromorphone, oxycodone, tramadol). Buprenorphine, alone of all the opioids, appears (at least in animal studies) to be devoid of effects on the immune system, whilst tramadol attenuates the immunosuppressive effects of surgery, again in animal studies. The relative effects of the opioids on the human immune system is only now being studied in detail, and how these effects relate to long-term administration of opioids to patients with chronic pain is not yet known.

7.3.6 **Respiratory effects**

Whilst the respiratory depressant effects of opioids given in acute pain are well recognized, respiratory depression is unusual when appropriate doses of oral or transdermal opioids are given to patients with chronic pain. The key safety mechanism is cautious and patient-specific dose titration, which is an important part of good practice in opioid prescription. Opioid-dependent respiratory depression can be revealed when patients maintained on long-acting opioids receive successful local nerve blockade. The explanation for this is that the respiratory depressant effects of opioids on the respiratory centre are balanced by nociceptive input. When that nociceptive input is interrupted, the brake on opioid-dependent respiratory depression is released, with potentially dangerous consequences.

There is also some anecdotal evidence that chronic opioid therapy can have effects on nocturnal respiratory control. Researchers performing polysomnography on patients thought to have obstructive sleep apnoea have noticed specific respiratory abnormalities associated with opioids. These abnormalities are:

- Prolonged apnoea and hypoxia, more severe during non-rapid eye movement (REM) sleep, compared to REM sleep.
- Ataxic breathing, characterized by irregular respiratory pauses and gasping without periodicity, present during non-REM sleep.
- Recurrent and unusually prolonged periods of obstructive hypoventilation, lasting at least 5 minutes, resulting in progressive severe hypoxaemia, and not present during REM sleep.

Whilst it is also known that 30% of patients on methadone maintenance programmes also have central sleep apnoea, it is not clear what the implications of these findings are for patients with chronic pain who are on long-term opioid treatment and who do not have obstructive sleep apnoea.

7.3.7 **Opioid-induced hyperalgesia**

As discussed in Chapter 2, prolonged opioid use can lead to desensitization (pharmacological tolerance). Conversely, prolonged use can also lead to abnormal pain sensitivity. This can take the form of hyperalgesia or allodynia. Distinguishing opioid-induced hyperalgesia (which may require a dose reduction or opioid switch) from disease progression or the development of tolerance (which may require a dose increase) can be difficult. However, opioid-induced hyperalgesia is usually characterized by pain that is more diffuse, less defined in quality, and in a wider spatial distribution than the pre-existing pain state. The mechanisms involved in this phenomenon are discussed more fully in Chapter 8.

7.3.8 **Pruritus and sweating**

Most of the data available on the dermatological side effects of opioids come from literature relating to opioid use in patients with cancer. The incidence of pruritus is variably reported, with one longitudinal study of 661 patients with cancer on transdermal fentanyl suggesting that 1.5% of patients suffer pruritus, but a meta-analysis of adverse effects of opioid therapy in non-cancer pain reported an incidence of 15%. The incidence is much higher when the epidural or intrathecal route is used. It is rarely a cause for cessation of treatment but, when it occurs, can be distressing and difficult to treat. Anecdotally, anti-histamines can be helpful, but there are no good data on which antihistamine to use. Sweating is thought to be mediated by either opioid-induced histamine release or by alterations in central thermoregulatory mechanisms. Again, anti-histamines can be a useful treatment as can anticholinergics, which inhibit exocrine sweat glands.

7.3.9 **Problem drug use**

Problem drug use in the setting of chronic non-cancer pain is uncommon but is the source of much anxiety in health professionals. Early recognition and referral to specialist services is essential. This topic is discussed more thoroughly in Chapter 14.

Key Reading

Abs R, Verhelst J, Maeyaert J, Van Buyten J, Opsomer F, Adriaensen H et al. (2000). Endocrine consequences of long-term intrathecal administration of opioids. *Journal of Clinical Endocrinology & Metabolism*, **85**, 2215–22.

Ballantyne J and Mao J (2003). Opioid therapy for chronic pain. *New England Journal of Medicine*, **349**, 1943–53.

Daniell HW (2008). Opioid endocrinopathy in women consuming prescribed sustained-action opioids for control of non-malignant pain. *Journal of Pain*, **9**, 28–36.

Driving and Vehicle Licensing Agency (n.d.). At a glance guide to the current medical guidelines (for medical professionals). Available from: http://www.dft.gov.uk/dvla/medical/aag.aspx [Accessed November 26, 2012].

Eriksen J, Sjørgren P, Bruera E, Elkholm O, and Rasmussen N (2006). Critical issues on opioids in chronic non-cancer pain: an epidemiological study. *Pain*, **125**, 172–9.

Grossman A (1983). Brain opiates and neuroendocrine function. *Clinics in Endocrinology and Metabolism*, **12**, 725–46.

Kalso E, Edwards JE, Moore A, and McQuay H (2004). Opioids in chronic non-cancer pain: systematic review of efficacy and safety. *Pain*, **112**, 372–80.

Katz N and Mazer NA (2009). The impact of opioids on the endocrine system. *Clinical Journal of Pain*, **25**, 170–5.

Kendall SE, Sjøgren P, and Pimenta CA (2010). The cognitive effects of opioids in chronic non-cancer pain. *Pain*, **150**, 225–30.

Kress HG and Kraft B (2005). Opioid medication and driving ability. *European Journal of Pain*, **9**, 141–4.

Mercadante S (1998). Pathophysiology and treatment of opioid-related myoclonus in cancer patients. *Pain*, **74**, 5–9.

Sacardote P (2006). Opioids and the immune system. *Palliative Medicine*, 20, S9–15.

Seyfried O and Hester J (2012). Opioids and endocrine dysfunction. *British Journal of Pain*, **6**, 17–24.

Vuong C, Van Uum SHM, O'Dell LE, Lutfy K, and Friedman TC (2010). The effects of opioids and opioid analogs on animal and human endocrine systems. *Endocrine Reviews*, **31**, 98–132.

Opioid-induced hyperalgesia

> Key points
> - Opioids have been shown in animal models to induce hyperalgesic states, particularly on withdrawal.
> - This phenomenon has also been seen in human experimental models, and it appears to occur in clinical practice.
> - The clinical importance of opioid-induced hyperalgesia in chronic pain remains to be fully evaluated.

43

8.1 Introduction

The concept of opioid-induced hyperalgesia (OIH) is evolving and is a current focus of active research activity. The principal idea seems counter-intuitive but stems from the paradoxical observation that opioids, under some circumstances, can cause modality-specific hyperalgesia and allodynia. There is a substantial base of animal model evidence that supports the concept of OIH. However, the human data are currently rather limited, as there are possible alternative explanations for the worsening of pain while on opioids such as progression of disease, development of a neuropathic element, or tolerance to the opioid regimen.

The idea that opioids might have pro-nociceptive actions, in addition to their analgesic activity, grew out of observations that hyperalgesia may occur in response to opioid withdrawal in both animal and human models. This has been seen following prolonged oral opioid therapy but also following short-term infusions of the potent, but ultra-short-acting, μ-OR agonist remifentanil. This has been replicated in humans, with expansion of an area of experimentally induced mechanical hyperalgesia following remifentanil administration. There is now evidence from animal studies that hyperalgesia may occur during opioid therapy, without the precipitant of a withdrawal of opioid treatment being necessary.

The animal data indicate that, after a period of acute or chronic opioid administration, there is a biphasic response consisting of analgesia, followed by a rebound hyperalgesic effect. This hyperalgesia may be mediated by sensitization of primary afferents, upregulation of glutamatergic transmission at a spinal level, increases in spinal dynorphin, and also descending facilitation from the brainstem. These biphasic actions of opioids are, at least, initiated through μ-ORs and appear distinct from the κ-OR-mediated hyperalgesia. Genetic analysis has linked this variability to differences in the β_2-adrenoceptor. It should be noted that relatively little work on OIH has been done in animal models of chronic pain, and there is no experimental evidence, animal or human, of OIH occurring during chronic opioid administration. A systematic review found little evidence for OIH in man outside of the setting of acute infusions studies of volunteers.

In man, OIH has been reported in the situations described in the following sections.

8.1.1 **In opioid withdrawal**

It has long been recognized that hyperalgesia accompanies opioid withdrawal reactions, and indeed it is a feature of withdrawal scoring systems. Several cross-sectional studies in former heroin addicts, maintained on a methadone programme, have shown them to have hyperalgesia to cold pressor testing when compared to a control group of former addicts not on a methadone programme. Some supportive data have been provided in a human experimental pain model where an induced area of hyperalgesia was increased in size after a 90-minute infusion of remifentanil.

8.1.2 **After acute administration of large doses of μ-agonists**

There are a number of case reports of patients receiving very large doses of opioids (commonly morphine) that induced a reversible, generalized allodynia. This was worsened in some cases by increasing the dose, and eased by switching the opioid. Interestingly, some of these effects appear resistant to opioid antagonists such as naloxone. Two studies of post-operative analgesic requirement have shown worse pain scores in patients receiving a large intra-operative dose of opioid. It is not clear, however, whether this is indicative of OIH or acute opioid tolerance. Furthermore, this finding was not verified in a follow-up study with similar methodology.

8.1.3 **Ultra-low-dose opioids**

There is a concept that opioids may produce hyperalgesia at very low doses, and analgesia at higher doses. There is some support for this concept from animal studies but little direct evidence from human studies. However, some patient studies have tested this idea indirectly, using co-administration of an opioid with a low dose of naloxone, in the hope that this will prevent the OIH and potentiate the analgesic effects. As yet, the findings from such studies are contradictory.

8.2 **Clinical relevance**

There are biologically plausible mechanisms by which opioids could produce hyperalgesia, particularly on withdrawal or during trough periods of continued dosing. However, as yet, patient studies have not provided an unequivocal demonstration that OIH is a clinically meaningful entity. A recent pilot study has been reported, which looked at patients with axial back pain before and after a 1-month course of opioids. The authors assessed the effect of remifentanil infusion on experimental pain measures (cold pressor test and heat pain threshold). This showed the development of both hyperalgesia and tolerance to the cold pressor test (but not heat pain) after 1 month of opioid administration. Importantly, however, the patients showed improvements in their pain scores when commenced on the opioids, leaving open the question of whether the OIH (and tolerance) was clinically significant.

Clinically, OIH is usually characterized by pain that has become more diffuse and less defined in quality and has a wider spatial distribution than the pre-existing pain state. The management of OIH typically involves a dose reduction or an opioid switch.

The rationale for opioid switching is little different to that used to avoid other opioid side effects. However, there is some emerging evidence from human pain studies that some opioids have different profiles as regard analgesia and anti-hyperalgesia. They have suggested that the pure μ-agonists may be less effective at attenuating secondary hyperalgesia than mixed opioid agonists/antagonists such as buprenorphine. Similar suggestions have been made in support of methadone because of its NMDA antagonist actions that may make it more effective in the treatment of sensitization. However, both these suggestions await validation in clinical trials.

It will be important to determine whether OIH is a meaningful entity in clinical practice. This is because opioid tolerance and OIH may appear similar, yet require entirely opposite treatment actions to provide relief. Thus, increasing the dose of opioid should treat tolerance, whereas the same course of action in OIH would be expected to exacerbate the problem. This issue is particularly relevant in the use of opioids for chronic non-malignant pains where, if OIH were shown to be a significant factor, it could swing the risk-benefit equation away from the use of opioids. It is clear that OIH could be a significant factor in the decision-making process around choosing to administer opioids (or indeed withdraw from) patients with chronic non-malignant pain, but clear and definitive studies will be required before this risk-benefit analysis can be calculated.

Key Reading

Angst MS and Clark JD (2006). Opioid-induced hyperalgesia: a qualitative systematic review. *Anesthesiology*, **104**, 570–87.

Chu LF, Clark DJ, and Angst MS (2006). Opioid tolerance and hyperalgesia in chronic pain patients after one month of oral morphine therapy: a preliminary prospective study. *Journal of Pain*, **7**, 43–8.

Colvin LA and Fallon MT (2010). Opioid-induced hyperalgesia: a clinical challenge. *British Journal of Anaesthesia*, **104**, 125–7.

Fishbain DA, Cole B, Lewis JE, Gao J, and Rosomoff RS (2009). Do opioids induce hyperalgesia in humans? An evidence-based structured review. *Pain Medicine*, **10**, 829–39.

Koppert W, Ihmsen H, Korber N, Wehrfritz A, Sittl R, Schmelz M et al. (2005). Different profiles of buprenorphine-induced analgesia and antihyperalgesia in a human pain model. *Pain*, **118**, 15–22.

Liang DY, Liao G, Wang J, Usuka J, Guo Y, Peltz G et al. (2006). A genetic analysis of opioid-induced hyperalgesia in mice. *Anesthesiology*, **104**, 1054–62.

Chapter 9

Contraindications, cautions, and drug interactions

Key points
- There are few absolute contraindications to opioid use.
- Renal and hepatic disease can result in significant alterations in drug handling, and dose reductions may be required.
- Opioids have a number of important drug interactions, which can result in altered pharmacokinetics or pharmacodynamics.

9.1 General considerations

An allergy to an opioid, or any of the pharmaceutical constituents of the preparation, is one of the few absolute contraindications to the use of opioids. Although allergies are uncommon, patients may be sensitive to opioid-induced histamine release. Patients who report an allergy to opioid medications usually describe recognized side effects of the drugs, which, if managed well, are not always a bar to opioid use.

The concomitant use of sedative drugs with opioids should be avoided if possible. Where this is not possible, patients must be warned that their psychomotor function is likely to be affected, and they should not drive or operate machinery. Patients who may benefit from opioid therapy but are currently abusing illicit substances or alcohol need expert assessment by teams experienced in managing such problems (see Chapter 14).

Patients often have anxieties regarding opioid treatment. A careful explanation of the treatment goals, possible adverse effects, and identifications of professional support during treatment is important.

A patient who remains reluctant to take opioids despite such reassurance is unlikely to comply with all aspects of treatment, and, in this situation, opioid therapy would be unwise.

9.2 Prescribing opioids for patients with medical comorbidity

9.2.1 Renal and hepatic disease

All the opioids in common use undergo some form of hepatic metabolism or renal excretion (see Chapter 2).

Morphine is metabolized in the liver to morphine-6-glucuronide, morphine-3-glucuronide, and normorphine. The glucuronide derivatives of morphine are renally excreted. Morphine-6-glucuronide is a potent μ-agonist and has analgesic effect. Much of the analgesic effect of morphine may be due to this metabolite. Morphine-3-glucuronide has been shown in animal studies to have effects on arousal. In a patient with hepatic or moderate to severe renal failure, the effect of morphine may be prolonged, and doses will need to be reduced or given less frequently. In severe hepatic failure, morphine may precipitate encephalopathy and should be avoided.

Fentanyl is also metabolized in the liver. N-dealkylation of the parent compound results in norfentanyl formation, and subsequent hydroxylation forms hydroxypropionyl derivatives. A small amount of the parent compound is excreted renally. Again, a reduced dose may be required in renal failure.

Tramadol undergoes hepatic demethylation, resulting in a number of metabolites, one of which, O-demethyl-tramadol, is active. Tramadol is highly renally excreted and is not recommended in severe renal failure. Patients with lesser degrees of renal or hepatic impairment will require a reduced or less frequent dose.

Buprenorphine undergoes significant first-pass metabolism. Transdermal or sublingual preparations avoid this phenomenon. Buprenorphine is dealkylated, then conjugated in the liver, and subsequently being excreted in bile into the gastrointestinal tract. There is no renal excretion of buprenorphine, and it is, therefore, safe to use in renal failure, with no dose adjustment.

Methadone has a very high volume of distribution and accumulates in the tissues with repeated doses. This accounts for its variable pharmacokinetics. It is chiefly metabolized in the liver, some of the drug and its metabolites being excreted by the kidneys, and some excreted by the liver into the intestinal tract. Renal and hepatic disease, however, do not seem to alter methadone clearance significantly.

9.2.2 **Respiratory disease**

All opioids are respiratory depressants, and, although respiratory depression in the setting of chronic, patient-specific oral/transdermal opioid therapy for pain is unusual, it is wise to be cautious in patients with significant pre-existing respiratory disease. Furthermore, opioids have been demonstrated to cause specific and profound alterations in respiratory performance during sleep in patients known to have obstructive sleep apnoea, which was discussed more fully in Chapter 7. Caution is advised when prescribing opioids for patients with this condition. The effects of long-term opioid therapy on sleep in otherwise healthy subjects are unknown, and data are required in this area.

Tramadol is unusual in that it has a number of modes of action and, at equianalgesic doses, probably causes less respiratory depression than the other opioids. Tramadol has little effect on hypercapnic respiratory drive, although it does affect hypoxic drive. Tramadol remains, however, the opioid of choice in patients where respiratory depression is a significant concern.

9.2.3 **Psychiatric disorders**

Whilst the presence of psychiatric comorbidity is not a contraindication to the use of opioids, it has to be recognized that opioids can be extremely dangerous or fatal in overdose. The interplay between mood and pain is complex, and, as discussed in Chapter 7, opioid analgesia can result in mood improvements. It is important to recognize that patients with mood disorder may take opioids to attenuate unpleasant thoughts and

Table 9.1 Opioid drug interactions		
Opioid	Interaction	Effects
Any opioid	Alcohol TCAs Antipsychotics Benzodiazepines	Increased CNS depressant effects. Enhanced reduction in psychomotor function
	MAOIs	CNS excitation or depression, avoid use within 2 weeks of stopping MAOIs (especially pethidine)
	Mexiletine	Reduced absorption of anti-arrhythmic
	Anti-emetics	Reduced anti-emetic effect
	Cimetidine	Reduced elimination and increased plasma concentration of opioid
	Antivirals	Increased plasma concentration of opioid (except methadone, see below)
	Cannabis	Increased sedative effect
Morphine	Rifampicin	Enhanced elimination of morphine
	Amitriptyline	Increased bioavailability of morphine
Tramadol	Coumarins	Enhanced anticoagulant effect
	SSRIs, TCAs, duloxetine	Enhanced risk of CNS toxicity
	Carbamazepine	Reduced analgesic effect
	Ondansetron	Reduced analgesic effect
	Selegiline	Possible increased risk of CNS toxicity
Methadone	Fluvoxamine	Increased plasma concentration of methadone
	Carbamazepine	Reduced plasma concentration of methadone
	Phenytoin Rifampicin	Enhanced metabolism of methadone, reduced effect, and risk of withdrawal
	Zidovudine	Increased plasma concentration of zidovudine
	Antivirals	Reduced plasma concentration of methadone
Buprenorphine	Other opioid (prescribed or illicit)	Partial agonist, may precipitate withdrawal

experiences, and it is important that this is evaluated when opioid therapy is being reviewed. Active suicidal intent needs urgent evaluation by mental health professionals, who need to be involved in the ongoing decision to prescribe opioids.

Prescribing for patients with a history of substance misuse is discussed in Chapter 14.

9.3 **Drug interactions**

Opioid analgesics have a number of important drug interactions that may require dose reductions, dose escalations, or avoidance of opioids altogether. The main interactions of interest to prescribers in the chronic pain setting are shown in Table 9.1.

Key Reading

Boger RH (2006). Renal impairment: a challenge for opioid treatment? The role of buprenorphine. *Palliative Medicine*, **20**, S17.

Joint Formulary Committee (2007). *British national formulary*. 53rd edn. British Medical Association and Royal Pharmaceutical Society of Great Britain, London.

Sasada M and Smith S (2003). *Drugs in anaesthesia and intensive care*. 3rd edn. Oxford Medical Publications, Oxford.

Chapter 10

Clinical use: back pain

> **Key points**
> - Back pain is common; few people need or request medical treatment; fewer still require opioid therapy.
> - Opioids are best used as part of a multimodal rehabilitation plan.
> - Evidence that opioids are effective analgesics for the treatment of low back pain and that they confer functional benefit comes from short-term studies.
> - Little is known about the long-term effectiveness of opioids in the management of low back pain.
> - Persistent pain following spinal surgery (failed back surgery syndrome) is difficult to manage: a trial of opioid therapy may be reasonable for this condition.

10.1 Epidemiology

In the developed world, chronic musculoskeletal pain is a common cause of disability, and low back pain is the most common painful musculoskeletal condition. Lifetime prevalence is estimated to be between 49% and 80%, and point prevalence between 12% and 35%. Back pain is currently the second commonest cause of sickness absence in the UK (mild to moderate mental health problems are the commonest cause). Reports of back pain increase with age and are commoner in women than men.

The majority of back pain episodes will be short and self-limiting, but a proportion of sufferers will go on to experience chronic and disabling symptoms. The result of this is a substantial financial burden to the UK, with costs to the Exchequer estimated at £12.3 billion annually. It is estimated that almost five million working days per year are lost as a result of back pain. Any treatment, if effective, has the potential to be of great benefit both to individual patients and the wider society.

10.2 Opioids as part of a multimodal treatment plan

Analgesic efficacy refers to the reduction in pain intensity that occurs as a result of analgesic use. However, chronic non-malignant back pain is a disorder that has complex biopsychosocial contributors. Effectiveness of treatment is usually judged not only by reductions in pain intensity but also by effects on the physical and psychological function, quality of life, and ability to work. Evidence for opioids in the treatment of chronic low back pain must, therefore, be assessed in these terms. If the use of opioids leads to a reduction in pain intensity, but at the cost of side effects that compromise wider goals of therapy, then they should not be used. Evidence supports a rehabilitative approach to chronic and subacute low back pain, and if opioids have a place at all in the management of chronic back pain, then it is only within a robust multimodal treatment plan.

10.3 Evidence for opioids in chronic back pain

Two consistent criticisms of the available literature are that studies tend to be of (relatively) short duration and focus mainly on reductions in pain intensity rather than examining the effects of opioids on wider function. The questions that need to be answered are:

1. Do opioids reduce pain intensity?
2. Do opioids aid physical rehabilitation?
3. Does opioid use result in improvements in physical and emotional well-being in the longer term?

10.3.1 Do opioids reduce pain intensity?

Most of the evidence in the literature comes from studies of opioids in patients with chronic pain of various types, amongst whom were a number who had back pain. One double-blinded, randomized controlled trial compared the effects of sustained-release morphine with benztropine (an active placebo chosen to aid blinding). The trial took, as its subjects, patients with chronic musculoskeletal pain, 44% of whom had low back pain. Initially, reasonable analgesia was seen (a reduction of around 25% in pain intensity), but, after 9 weeks of treatment, this effect was less marked. There were no improvements in physical or psychological function. The study did not stratify response to therapy as a function of the site of pain, but, assuming the response of the study group as a whole was representative of the response of those patients with low back pain, this study supported the utility of opioids in reducing pain intensity in the short to medium term (days to weeks). One randomized, double-blinded, placebo-controlled study has been conducted in patients with 'osteoarthritis pain', half of which were classified as having 'back or neck pain'. The 2-week trial of oxycodone modified release versus placebo showed a dose-dependent reduction in pain intensity and improvements in mood, sleep, and quality of life. The majority of patients proceeded to a 6-month, open-label phase, which showed continuing benefit, with little evidence of dose escalation.

Tapentadol gained FDA approval in the US for use in moderate to severe acute pain in 2008, and MHRA approval in the UK in February 2011. There is, therefore, currently little evidence on which to base conclusions about its long-term efficacy in the chronic pain population. We have to extrapolate data from short-term studies and, therefore, any conclusions are open to challenge.

Low back pain is a complex socio-economic and clinical phenomenon. It can show nociceptive and neuropathic components, and treatment with drugs from one pharmacological class can, at best, be partially effective and often limited by dose-limiting side effects. As a mixed-pain state, there is theoretical validity in the use of an analgesic with a wide range of action in its management. Tapentadol has a dual mode of action, being an agonist at the μ-OR and an inhibitor of norepinephrine re-uptake mechanisms. The contribution of these two mechanisms to the analgesic effect of tapentadol is stable over time and from patient to patient, unlike the superficially similar drug tramadol.

We have some evidence from short-term studies (up to 12–15 weeks in length) that, at equianalgesic doses to oxycodone, adequate to result in a meaningful reduction in pain intensity, tapentadol is better tolerated than oxycodone. In one such study, around half of the number of patients taking tapentadol withdrew from the study due to an adverse effect, compared to those taking oxycodone. Another study has evaluated the longer-term safety of tapentadol in this patient population over a period of a year. Pain intensity was assessed as a secondary outcome measure, and a consistent reduction in pain was shown over the duration of the study.

Although the evidence is still modest and there are, as yet, no long-term studies of tapentadol in the treatment of chronic low back pain with pain intensity as a primary outcome measure, there is preliminary evidence to suggest that tapentadol may have utility in this patient group.

All of the other reported trials are either open-label or non-randomized or both, or retrospective reviews. One such trial had three treatment arms. Patients with back pain were randomized to either a non-steroidal anti-inflammatory drug, fixed-dose oxycodone, or sustained-release morphine, with additional oxycodone titrated to pain intensity. The trial is interesting, as it was conducted over the course of a year, with a titration phase, an experimental phase, and a tapering-off phase, mimicking clinical practice. The trial was blinded neither to the patient nor to the investigators, so the results have to be viewed in that context, but nevertheless patients in the titrated group reported significantly less pain and improved mood. There were no significant differences in levels of activity or sleep. Interestingly, although the patients in the titrated group were using an immediate-release preparation, there was no notable tendency for the opioid requirement to escalate during the course of the study. Another trial followed patients treated with a long-acting opioid for an average of 32 months. Although this trial was neither blinded nor placebo-controlled, patients showed a reduction in the Pain Numerical Rating Scale score and the Oswestry Low Back Disability score.

More recently, a systematic review of trials of opioid treatment for chronic back pain has been published. This review identified six trials where the comparator was a placebo or a non-opioid medication, and nine trials where different opioids or different doses of the same opioid were used as comparators. The review concluded that there is weak evidence for the short-term (less than 16 weeks) use of opioids in chronic back pain but no good evidence for longer-term use.

10.3.2 Do opioids aid rehabilitation?

Evidence for the effectiveness of opioids in facilitating physical rehabilitation is scarce. What evidence there is comes from observations that opioids improve exercise tolerance in experimental settings. Some authorities have inferred from this that opioids are likely to be useful as part of a multimodal, exercise-based rehabilitation programme for patients with subacute low back pain. This assertion has yet to be held up to rigorous scientific scrutiny, and opioids should be used with caution in this group of patients.

10.3.3 Does opioid use result in improvements in physical and emotional well-being in the long term?

Evidence for sustained functional improvement as a consequence of opioid therapy is from long-term observational studies and a number of shorter trials that are either non-randomized, non-blinded or non-placebo-controlled. There is some experimental evidence, however, that opioids can result in improvements in physical function.

Evidence for long-term utility of opioid therapy in treating back pain comes from ret-rospective reviews and case series. More recently, a large cross-sectional study based on the 2000 Danish Health and Morbidity Study has been reported. Denmark has an extremely high rate of opioid use, with 3% of the population using opioids on a regular or continuous basis. Of the 19% of people who reported chronic pain (defined as pain present for more than 6 months), 12% were using opioids. Amongst this group of patients, opioid use was associated with poor self-rated health, poor employment status, low quality of life, and high levels of health care consumption, even when dif-ferences in pain intensity were taken into account. Although the responses were not stratified by site of pain, a large proportion had chronic back pain, and the conclusions are reasonably applicable to this patient group.

10.4 **Failed back surgery syndrome**

Patients who have back pain following one or more spinal surgical interventions pose particular clinical challenges. Around 2,000 individuals per year in the UK will enter the somewhat unsatisfactorily labelled diagnostic group of failed back surgery syndrome (FBSS). FBSS is difficult to manage, with less than a third of patients being helped by spe-cialist pain services. For those who derive some benefit, improvements are modest. It is often not possible to define why symptoms persist, but patients will often present with components of both nociceptive and neuropathic pain. Radicular symptoms may per-sist in up to 10% of patients following spinal surgery, either because of nerve damage from the original insult (e.g. disc prolapse or spondylophytic compression) or because of neural scarring as a consequence of surgical intervention. Patients with FBSS have often spent much time in contact with health care services that have failed to help them, with the inevitable consequences of the frequently repeated cycle of optimism that submission to surgery will provide a definitive fix for symptoms, followed by dis-appointment and regret that they are left worse off than where they started. Little is written about opioid therapy in these patients: much of the literature relates to invasive interventions such as spinal cord stimulation and intrathecal therapy. Given that these patients have symptoms that have been worsened by surgery, it seems reasonable to explore non-surgical options, including opioid therapy where possible, always in the context of a comprehensive pain management plan, aimed at improvement in function and quality of life.

10.5 **Conclusion**

Short-term opioid treatment of chronic back pain is supported by the available data, but long-term recommendations are hampered by a lack of clear guidance from lon-gitudinal studies. There is little guidance in the literature about the use of opioids for FBSS, although this challenging clinical situation probably justifies a trial of strong opioid as part of a pain management plan. Although there is evidence from a large cross-sectional population study that opioid use may be associated with poor self-reported health, unemployment, and high levels of health care use, large population studies will always fail to identify individual success stories, and this is particularly the case for a con-dition such as chronic low back pain where sufferers have heterogenous aetiologies and presentations. All clinicians who prescribe opioids for chronic non-cancer pain know of patients who have had their lives changed for the better. Such experience must be balanced by the knowledge that opioid use is associated with significant adverse effects, and that any benefits may be marginal.

Key Reading

Bartleson J (2002). Evidence for and against the use of opioid analgesics for chronic non-malignant low back pain: a review. *Pain Medicine*, **3**, 260–71.

Buynak R, Shapiro DY, Okamoto A, Van Hove I, Rauschkolb C, Steup A et al. (2010). Efficacy and safety of tapentadol extended release for the management of chronic low back pain: results of a prospective, randomized, double-blind, placebo- and active-controlled Phase III study. *Expert Opinion on Pharmacotherapy*, **11**, 1787–804.

Chief Medical Officer (2009). Pain: breaking through the barrier, 2008 annual report. Available from: http://www.dh.gov.uk/prod_consum_dh/groups/dh_digitalassets/documents/digitalasset/dh_096233.pdf [Accessed November 26, 2012].

Eriksen J, Sjøgren P, Bruera E, Ekholm O, and Rasmussen N (2006). Critical issues on opioids in chronic non-cancer pain: an epidemiological study. *Pain*, **125**, 172–9.

Jamison RN, Raymond SA, Slawsby EA, Nedeljkovic SS, and Katz NP (1998). Opioid therapy for chronic non-cancer back pain: a randomized prospective study. *Spine*, **23**, 2591–600.

Martell B, O'Connor P, Kerns R, Becker WC, Morales KH, Kosten TR et al. (2007). Systematic review: opioid treatment for chronic back pain: prevalence, efficacy, and association with addiction. *Annals of Internal Medicine*, **146**, 116–27.

Moulin DE, Iezzi A, Amireh R, Sharpe WK, Boyd D, and Merskey H (1996). Randomised trial of oral morphine for chronic non-cancer pain. *Lancet*, **347**, 143–7.

Portenoy R (1989). Opioid therapy. In: SD Tollinson, ed. *Interdisciplinary rehabilitation of low back pain*, pp. 137–57. Williams and Wilkins, Baltimore.

Talbot L (2003). Failed back surgery syndrome. *BMJ*, **327**, 985–6.

Wild JE, Grond S, Kuperwasser B, Gilbert J, McCann B, Lange B et al. (2010). Long-term safety and tolerability of tapentadol extended release for the management of chronic low back pain or osteoarthritis pain. *Pain Practice*, **10**, 416–27.

Chapter 11

Clinical use: pain associated with osteoarthritis

Key points

- Osteoarthritis is a progressive disease. Symptoms can include severe pain and loss of function.
- Opioids are effective analgesics, although the magnitude of the effect may be small.
- On the basis of the available evidence, widespread use of strong opioids cannot be recommended.
- With careful patient selection, however, certain patients may derive analgesic and functional benefit.

11.1 Introduction

Osteoarthritis can be a progressive disease of synovial joints. It is characterized by destruction of articular surfaces and remodelling of subchondral bone. Osteoarthritis is the result of a disturbance of the normal balance between cartilage production and loss. Cartilage breakdown, the result of the actions of proteolytic enzymes such as the matrix metalloproteinases, is accompanied by an increase in the activity of chondrocytes attempting tissue repair.

The most commonly affected joints are the interphalangeal joints of the hands, knees, and hips, and the facet joints of the cervical and lumbar spine. Usual symptoms include pain, swelling, stiffness, and loss of function.

The diagnosis of osteoarthritis is made on a combination of clinical features and radiographic evidence. X-rays have to be interpreted with some caution, however, as considerable pathological changes may occur before radiographs become abnormal, and, furthermore, osteoarthritis seen on X-rays may be completely asymptomatic.

Some osteoarthritis, e.g. of the hip or knee, responds well to operative treatment. When symptoms are the result of osteoarthritis in joints not amenable to surgery, or where patient comorbidities preclude surgery, treatment is palliative. Opioids can be a part of successful symptomatic management.

Much of the evidence regarding the symptomatic treatment of chronic back pain, presented in Chapter 10, has relevance in osteoarthritis. There is incomplete crossover, however, as osteoarthritis pain refers to pain arising from the damaged articular surfaces, whereas back pain can arise not only from the synovial joints of the spine but also from discs, spinal nerves, paraspinal muscles, and other spinal structures.

Osteoarthritis is an age-related condition. When considering prescribing strong opioids to elderly patients, it is vital to assess the balance of benefits and adverse effects carefully on a patient-by-patient basis.

11.2 **Evidence for effectiveness of opioids in the treatment of osteoarthritis pain**

There have been a number of trials specifically addressing the opioid responsiveness of osteoarthritis pain. One trial randomized 107 patients with persistent moderate to severe pain, uncontrolled with standard therapy (non-steroidal anti-inflammatory drugs (NSAIDs), paracetamol, and/or short-acting opioids) to either controlled-release oxycodone or placebo. Over the study period of 90 days, those patients taking the active drug reported statistically significant reductions in pain intensity and improved measures of physical functioning. The magnitude of these improvements, however, was small (in the case of pain intensity, approximately 1 point on an 11-point scale), although patients reported much higher levels of satisfaction with medication when taking the opioid compared to the placebo. Another study randomized patients to receive transdermal fentanyl or placebo. Although this study demonstrated a small improvement in mean pain scores at 1–3 weeks, this was not sustained past 4 weeks. The WOMAC (Western Ontario and McMaster Universities Osteoarthritis) index, a measurement of physical function, also improved. The drug manufacturers, who funded the trial, were involved in the study design and statistical analysis.

A recent meta-analysis of randomized, placebo-controlled trials of pharmacotherapeutic interventions in osteoarthritic knee pain identified five trials where the active drug was a strong opioid, and one trial where the active drug was codeine. The pooled data from 1,057 patients showed that, over the short term, there was a statistically significant reduction in pain. The magnitude of that analgesic effect, however, was only 10.5 mm on a 0–100 mm visual analogue scale (VAS). The applicability of these findings, however, is limited by the fact that the authors failed to distinguish between opioids and made no assessment as to the appropriateness of the opioid doses used in the included trials.

The use of tramadol in osteoarthritic pain has been the subject of a Cochrane review. Eleven trials were identified, all of which were of good methodological quality. The pooled data indicate that, whilst there is good evidence that tramadol is an effective analgesic in osteoarthritis, the magnitude of that effect is small, corresponding to 12.5 mm on a VAS. The number needed to harm (NNTH; the number of patients needed to be treated for one to suffer an adverse effect) for minor adverse effects was similar to the number needed to benefit, although the NNTH is significantly reduced if there is a slow upward dose titration during the initial phase of treatment. The use of tramadol also confers a small beneficial effect on function, equivalent to 0.32 points on the 0–10 WOMAC index of function.

As noted in Chapter 10, we currently have little evidence concerning the prolonged use of tapentadol. A number of phase III studies have shown reductions in pain after 12–15 weeks of treatment. The mean reduction in pain in one paper, using data from pooled phase III studies, was of a magnitude of around 2.5 points on an 11-point Numerical Rating Scale (NRS); this represented a statistically significantly greater pain reduction than both oxycodone controlled release and placebo, although the reduction was modest. In addition, a greater proportion of patients treated with tapentadol reached the threshold of 30% improvement in NRS in comparison with those treated with oxycodone, the usual pain reduction that is held to be clinically significant.

One could argue that the oxycodone dose was non-equianalgesic, and the patients in the active control group were underdosed. One has to look at the adverse events to determine whether the risk-benefit ratio for tapentadol is significantly different to its comparators, and indeed, in this study, despite the oxycodone being less efficacious, more patients withdrew due to adverse events in the oxycodone groups than in the tapentadol groups. This is in harmony with studies that show improved gastrointestinal tolerability of tapentadol, compared to oxycodone at doses deemed to be equianalgesic either through pre-clinical animal studies or measures of efficacy in the human pain population.

Although data are limited, tapentadol holds the promise of modest analgesic activity, with improved tolerability in comparison to oxycodone. We will have to await longer-term studies comparing tapentadol to different comparators to be clear where it sits in the expanding range of opioid and dual-mechanism drugs that are available to us.

11.3 **Conclusion**

There is good evidence that strong opioids, including tramadol, have analgesic efficacy in osteoarthritic pain. The magnitude of this benefit, however, is small and the number needed to treat high (around 6). Little is known about the long-term effectiveness of opioids in improving analgesia or function. Given that the patient population with osteoarthritis is predominantly elderly, in whom opioid side effects can be expected to be more severe, a careful assessment needs to be made of the potential benefits and risks prior to starting a trial of strong opioids.

Key Reading

Afilalo M, Etropolski MS, Kuperwasser B, Kelly K, Okamoto A, Van Hove I et al. (2010). Efficacy and safety of tapentadol extended release compared with oxycodone controlled release for the management of moderate to severe chronic pain related to osteoarthritis of the knee: a randomized, double-blind, placebo- and active-controlled phase III study. *Clinical Drug Investigation*, **30**, 489–505.

Bjordal JM, Klovning A, Ljunggren AE, and Slørdal L (2007). Short-term efficacy of pharmacotherapeutic interventions in osteoarthritic knee pain: a meta-analysis of placebo-controlled trials. *European Journal of Pain*, **11**, 125–38.

Cepeda MS, Camargo F, Zea C, and Valencia L (2006). Tramadol for osteoarthritis (review). *Cochrane Database of Systematic Reviews*, CD005522.

Hale M, Upmalis D, Okamoto A, Lange C, and Rauschkolb C (2009). Tolerability of tapentadol immediate release in patients with lower back pain or osteoarthritis of the hip or knee over 90 days: a randomized, double-blind study. *Current Medical Research & Opinion*, **25**, 1095–104.

Lange B, Kuperwasser B, Okamoto A, Steup A, Häufel T, Ashworth J et al. (2010). Efficacy and safety of tapentadol prolonged release for chronic osteoarthritis pain and low back pain. *Advances in Therapy*, **27**, 381–99.

Langford R, McKenna F, Ratcliffe S, Vojtassak J, and Richarz U (2006). Transdermal fentanyl for improvement of pain and functioning in osteoarthritis. *Arthritis and Rheumatism*, **54**, 1829–37.

Markenson JA, Croft J, Zhang PG, and Richards P (2005). Treatment of persistent pain associated with osteoarthritis with controlled release oxycodone tablets in a randomized controlled clinical trial. *Clinical Journal of Pain*, **21**, 524–35.

Wild JE, Grond S, Kuperwasser B, Gilbert J, McCann B, Lange B et al. (2010). Long-term safety and tolerability of tapentadol extended release for the management of chronic low back pain or osteoarthritis pain. *Pain Practice*, **10**, 416–27.

Clinical use: neuropathic pain

- Opioids can be useful in treating neuropathic pain. There are theoretical reasons why neuropathic pain may show reduced sensitivity to opioid therapy.
- Morphine, oxycodone, and tramadol have the best published evidence to support their use in the treatment of neuropathic pain.
- Opioids may have a role in reducing other pain sensations such as static or dynamic allodynia.

12.1 Introduction

Neuropathic pain was previously thought to be refractory to opioid therapy. In an influential study, a small number of patients with mixed nociceptive and neuropathic pain were treated with boluses of intravenous morphine or saline placebo and observed for a short period (less than an hour). Only three out of the 12 patients with neuropathic pain reported significant pain relief, and this led to the conclusion that neuropathic pain was unresponsive to opioids. This paper has subsequently been criticized, as the majority of patients entering the trial were previous opioid non-responders.

In 1991, the notion of non-responsiveness of neuropathic pain to opioids was challenged. A trial was published demonstrating that, compared to saline placebo, intravenous morphine reduced the intensity of the pain of post-herpetic neuralgia, at least under experimental conditions. The following year, a case series using morphine patient-controlled analgesia (PCA) patients, with either nociceptive or neuropathic pain, gave results that seemed to imply that some neuropathic pains are opioid-responsive, independent of the opioid effects on mood. Because of the unpredictable response of neuropathic pain to opioids, the paper recommended intravenous testing to determine opioid responsiveness prior to starting long-term therapy. The validity of intravenous opioid testing as a predictor of longer-term efficacy has now been challenged.

Throughout the 1990s, further studies were published suggesting that neuropathic pain is not inherently unresponsive to opioid therapy, and a consensus has grown that, for certain patients under certain conditions, opioids can be helpful (see Section 12.2 Evidence for efficacy of opioids in neuropathic pain). It remains a widely held view that neuropathic pain, whilst demonstrably effectively treated by opioids, is relatively opioid-resistant when compared to nociceptive pain, although this is not supported by results of randomized controlled trials of opioids in these two types of pain condition. There are, however, a number of scientific observations that shed further light on the neurophysiology of the opioid system in health and in neuropathic pain states, which, if extrapolated to the clinical setting, might suggest that neuropathic pain may show reduced sensitivity to opioid therapy.

Opioids are thought to have actions at both spinal and supra-spinal levels. Opioid receptors are present both presynaptically and post-synaptically at the termination of large nociceptive C-fibres in the substantia gelatinosa in the superficial dorsal horn. Activation of presynaptic opioid receptors leads to the opening of potassium channels in the presynaptic membrane, and the resultant calcium flux inhibits neurotransmitter release. Activation of post-synaptic opioid receptors both hyperpolarizes the post-synaptic membrane, therefore making it less sensitive to depolarization in response to neurotransmitter release, and disinhibits inhibitory interneurones. Both these effects lead to a reduction in onward nociceptive transmission.

The balance of pro-nociceptive and anti-nociceptive influences is altered following nerve injury. ORs are synthesized in the cell bodies of afferent neurones in the dorsal root ganglion and migrate to peripheral and central nerve terminals. Axonal transport is reduced, following complete or partial nerve injury, and consequently a reduction in opioid receptor density in the dorsal horn occurs. Additionally, calcium channel activity, essential for neurotransmitter release, is upregulated following nerve injury, further shifting the balance towards pain transmission. The role of the NMDA receptor system in generating the phenomenon of wind-up and long-term potentiation in models of nerve injury is well recognized and explains the fact that opioids and NMDA antagonists demonstrate potentiation of each other's actions.

Further pro-nociceptive activity may be the result of the actions of cholecystokinin (CCK) on the opioid system. In non-pathological states, primary afferent neurones are devoid of CCK receptors. Nerve injury induces the production of CCK receptors in peripheral nerves, and CCK appears to function as an anti-opioid peptide. CCK antagonists have been shown to be analgesics in models of neuropathic pain, and, furthermore, they appear to re-establish opioid responsiveness in those models.

Although the mode of central anti-nociceptive action of opioids is poorly understood, opioid receptors are known to exist in brainstem and midbrain nuclei such as the raphe nuclei, the periaqueductal grey, and the locus coeruleus. Higher centres, including the medial thalamus and the insular, temporal, and prefrontal cortices, also demonstrate opioid binding. Functional imaging studies have revealed a bilateral reduction in exogenous opioid binding in these higher structures in patients with chronic peripheral neuropathic pain, possibly reflecting endogenous opioid release and subsequent receptor site occupation. Importantly, patients with central post-stroke pain show a more marked and unilateral reduction in exogenous opioid binding, contralateral to the painful side, in areas exceeding the lesion sites. This seems likely to represent a specific loss or inactivation of opioid receptors in regions interconnected to the zone of neuronal death and may explain the reduced opioid sensitivity seen in patients with centrally mediated pain.

12.2 Evidence for efficacy of opioids in neuropathic pain

Neuropathic pain is defined by the International Association for the Study of Pain as pain caused by a lesion or disease of the somatosensory nervous system. This definition encompasses a number of disorders, including so-called nociceptive neuropathic pain arising as a result of activation of the nervi-nervorum around nerve trunks due to mechanical or chemical irritation (e.g. sciatica) to central post-stroke pain, or deafferentation pain resulting from sectioning of peripheral nerve fibres. Studies tend to be carried out using highly selected patient groups in clearly defined diagnostic categories (e.g. post-herpetic neuralgia, painful diabetic neuropathy, trigeminal neuralgia), which, by definition, have pain arising as a result of a common mechanism or combination of mechanisms. Even when a trial has flawless methodology, this makes the application of results to everyday clinical practice and other patient groups difficult. As neuropathic pains of any aetiology can have a number of common symptoms, such as spontaneous burning pain or static or dynamic mechanical allodynia, some experts now advocate that treatment and scientific investigation should proceed using a symptom-based approach to patient selection.

The use of opioids in the treatment of neuropathic pain has been the subject of two meta-analyses performed by the Cochrane Collaboration. One reviews full opioid agonists, and the other evaluates evidence relating to the weak μ-OR agonist and monoaminergic drug tramadol. Both of these reviews concentrate primarily on spontaneous pain. The use of opioids in the management of evoked neuropathic pain will be considered separately. There are no high-quality data relating to the long-term efficacy of μ-agonists for the management of neuropathic pain. The most reliable data available are from trials that have studied opioid therapy for up 10 weeks. Although some of the published trials have recruited patients with a single diagnosis, a number of them involved patients with neuropathic pain of diverse aetiology. The results of these trials may, therefore, be more applicable to a wider clinical practice.

12.2.1 **Morphine**

A number of high-quality randomized controlled trials have been published, comparing morphine against other anti-neuropathic pain medications or placebo. In the majority of these trials, morphine was given intravenously or intramuscularly, and conclusions were based on short-term follow-up, i.e. hours or days. One early trial randomized patients to receive high concentration (30 mg/ml) or low concentration (10 mg/ml) of morphine via a PCA device. Boluses were of 0.05 ml, giving doses of 1.5 mg and 0.5 mg, respectively. Patients judged to have nociceptive pain responded better than those with neuropathic pain, but half of those with neuropathic pain showed a good response. In all patients, the response to the high concentration was better than to the low concentration. Another trial of intravenous morphine deserves special mention, as it recruited patients with central pain, resulting from cerebrovascular accidents or spinal cord injury. The 15 subjects were randomized to either intravenous morphine boluses or inert placebo. Morphine significantly reduced dynamic allodynia but not other evoked pains. There was no clear effect of morphine on spontaneous pain.

Four published double-blinded, randomized controlled trials have studied morphine given orally over a longer period (weeks). One of these trials tested oral sustained-release morphine sulphate (MST®) versus placebo in 12 patients with phantom limb pain. The trial had a crossover design, with two phases, each of 4 weeks. Patients received either MST® followed by placebo or placebo followed by MST®. When taking MST®, 42% of patients reported more than 50% analgesia, compared to 8% reporting more than 50% analgesia when taking placebo. Conclusions from this trial are tempered by the knowledge that, despite efforts to ensure blinding, both researchers and patients could reliably identify the active treatment phase. Another trial compared the effects of morphine, a tricyclic antidepressant (TCA), and placebo on 76 patients with post-herpetic neuralgia, in three phases of 8 weeks each. Similar numbers of patients reported pain relief with opioids and TCAs, compared to placebo (38% and 32% versus 8%, respectively). A different group of patients responded to opioids or TCAs, implying that they work by different and independent mechanisms. A third trial reported significant pain relief only when morphine was used in combination with the anti-epileptic gabapentin. Interestingly, this trial failed to show any benefit of gabapentin on neuropathic pain when used alone. A fourth trial took, as its subjects, patients with complex regional pain syndrome type 1 who were successfully treated with spinal cord stimulation. Patients were instructed to turn off their stimulator and then received sustained-release morphine (90 mg per day), carbamazepine, or placebo. There was no beneficial effect of morphine at the dose specified, although patients reported significant analgesia with carbamazepine.

12.2.2 Oxycodone

Oxycodone has been the active treatment in three high-quality randomized controlled trials. The first of these trials, published almost a decade ago, randomized patients with post-herpetic neuralgia to controlled-release oxycodone (initially, 20 mg per day, increasing to a maximum of 60 mg per day) or placebo, each for a treatment period of 4 weeks, in a crossover design. Of 50 enrolled patients, 38 completed the study protocol. Oxycodone was superior to placebo in relieving steady pain, allodynia, and paroxysmal spontaneous pain. One of the authors of this study subsequently published a controlled trial, randomizing patients with painful diabetic neuropathy to an escalating dose of controlled-release oxycodone (20–40 mg oxycodone per day) or benztropine (an active placebo) in a crossover protocol. This study design was chosen to help minimize patient and researcher unblinding as a result of side effects attributable to the active treatment arm. The results revealed a clinically significant reduction in background and spontaneous pain, and improved measures of quality of life in patients taking oxycodone. Another randomized controlled trial comparing oxycodone and inactive placebo in diabetic neuropathy has shown similar results, albeit of smaller magnitude. Of note, however, is that the treatment arms lasted no longer than 4 weeks in any of these trials.

12.2.3 Fentanyl

One randomized controlled trial compared the analgesic effect of intravenous fentanyl with an active placebo (diazepam) and an inert placebo (saline) in a group of 53 patients with mixed neuropathic pain. Patients received an infusion of fentanyl (5 mcg/kg/hour) or placebo for 5 hours and were studied for a further 3 hours following cessation of the infusion. Maximum pain intensity and pain unpleasantness were reduced during the fentanyl infusion but not during placebo. Of the 50 patients completing the study, 48 went on to take part in an open-label, non-randomized trial of transdermal fentanyl, which was reported separately. Of the 48 patients, 18 stopped treatment early due to lack of pain relief. Thirty patients completed the 12-week trial period, 18 of them reporting moderate or substantial pain relief. There are no blinded, randomized studies of transdermal fentanyl for neuropathic pain.

12.2.4 Methadone

Methadone is a μ-OR agonist that also demonstrates inhibition of monoamine re-uptake and antagonism of the action of glutamate, the endogenous ligand at NMDA receptors. This latter property is important, as NMDA activity has been implicated in the development of opioid tolerance, and also the development of 'wind-up'-type symptoms (common in neuropathic pain) and long-term potentiation, which results from the high rates of ectopic discharge seen following nerve injury. In animal models of neuropathic pain, NMDA antagonists are anti-nociceptive and strongly potentiate the action of opioids when they are administered together. Despite this, there has been only one trial of high quality, lasting a total of 40 days, which compared two sequential doses of methadone or placebo. Thirty-three patients with mixed neuropathic pain were invited to participate, of whom 19 accepted. One patient subsequently withdrew from the trial during phase I (low-dose methadone). Six of the remaining 17 patients failed to complete the trial, leaving only 11 of the original 33 patients in the final analysis. Although the results may have little validity on an intention-to-treat basis, this trial demonstrated statistically significant improvements in pain scores at the higher dose of 20 mg per day, but improvements at the lower dose of 10 mg per day failed to reach statistical significance. Despite its intuitive appeal, therefore, there is no clear evidence that methadone is superior to other μ-agonists. Methadone can be useful in the management of morphine-induced hyperalgesia, which may have a mechanistic commonality with neuropathic pain, but, on a practical level, the use of methadone is complicated by highly variable pharmacokinetics from patient to patient that makes dose titration difficult.

12.2.5 **Tramadol**

Tramadol is a drug that has weak μ-opioid effect and a weak monoaminergic effect. Its use in neuropathic pain has recently been the subject of a systematic review, which identified six high-quality, double-blinded, randomized trials. One trial randomized 131 patients with painful diabetic neuropathy to receive either oral tramadol or inert placebo. At day 42, patients in the treatment group had significantly lower pain intensity. Secondary outcome measures included physical and social functioning, which were also better in the tramadol group than the placebo group. A second trial randomized 127 patients with post-herpetic neuralgia to two parallel study groups: one group receiving tramadol 100–300 mg per day, the other an inert placebo. Both groups showed a clinically significant reduction in pain measured on a VAS, with the reduction more marked in the tramadol group. The time from onset of post-herpetic neuralgia to inclusion in the study was not longer than 12 months in any patient, so the general improvement in symptoms may have been related to the natural history of the disease.

All the double-blinded, randomized controlled trials, using tramadol as the active treatment, have been performed in patients with peripheral neuropathic pain, and, in this group of patients, it appears that it is an effective treatment. There is no clear evidence, however, that it is more effective than morphine or oxycodone. Tramadol has less effect on the hypercapnic respiratory response than morphine, and, in addition, it appears to be less constipating. It may, therefore, have a role.

12.2.6 **Tapentadol**

Tapentadol is a novel analgesic with a dual mode of action; firstly, it is a weak agonist at the μ-OR, and, secondly, it is a selective norepinephrine re-uptake inhibitor. Its anti-nociceptive and anti-hyperalgesic effects are partially retained in μ-OR knock-out mice, confirming the importance of the second of these two mechanisms to its overall analgesic action. Like the TCAs and the superficially similar drug tramadol, it has a mode of action that is associated with efficacy in neuropathic pain states. In a study utilizing the spinal nerve ligation rat model of neuropathic pain, tapentadol showed a dose-dependent increase in mechanical paw withdrawal thresholds, a behavioural correlate of mechanical allodynia in human subjects with chronic neuropathic pain. In this study, tapentadol showed synergism when used in combination with pregabalin, an anticonvulsant with action at the alpha-2-delta subunit of voltage-gated calcium channels. The same group showed a reduction in heat allodynia in a mouse model of diabetic neuropathy, with no such effect seen in non-diabetic animals. One study in human subjects has shown a statistical improvement in pain scores in patients with painful diabetic neuropathy treated with tapentadol, compared to those treated with placebo. However, when compared with placebo, treatment with tapentadol only yielded an average improvement of 1.3 points on an 11-point (0–10) NRS, which, although statistically significant, does not reach the 3-point improvement usually taken to be indicative of clinical significance. We await further studies to determine whether the beneficial effects seen in animal models, and the modest benefits seen in the human study described above, are indicative of wider efficacy in patients with chronic neuropathic pain.

12.2.7 **Buprenorphine**

Buprenorphine is a potent opioid that demonstrates partial agonism at μ-OR, and antagonism at the δ-and κ-OR. It is available as both a sublingual tablet and as a transdermal patch. There is evidence from animal studies that buprenorphine may have additional mechanisms of action, not possessed by other opioids that may be relevant to the action of the drug in neuropathic pain. However, there is limited evidence of clinical effectiveness in the setting of chronic neuropathic pain. One trial of 21 post-thoracotomy patients with persisting thoracic pain 1 month after surgery examined responses to varying doses of intravenous buprenorphine. Pain thresholds to electrical stimulation were measured, and the authors concluded that spontaneous and evoked neuropathic pains are both reduced by buprenorphine. Another trial studied the effect of transdermal buprenorphine on mixed cancer and non-cancer nociceptive and neuropathic pains. Patients were randomized to receive low-, medium-, or high-dose buprenorphine, or placebo. Patients receiving the low- or medium-dose buprenorphine reported significantly higher response rates than with placebo, but, interestingly, this was not seen in patients receiving the high-dose buprenorphine. Buprenorphine has some theoretical advantages over other opioids, but, as yet, there is no convincing evidence of long-term efficacy in neuropathic pain.

12.2.8 **Levorphanol**

Levorphanol is a μ-agonist that is approximately 30 times more potent than morphine. Like methadone, it demonstrates antagonism at the NMDA receptor and inhibits biogenic amine re-uptake and thus has theoretical advantages in neuropathic pain. It is currently not commercially available in the UK, but it has been studied in chronic peripheral and central neuropathic pain syndromes (see Section 12.3 Evoked neuropathic pain; Section 12.4 Central pain).

12.3 **Evoked neuropathic pain**

A recent systematic review examined the evidence for the use of opioids in evoked neuropathic pain. Evoked pain, comprising static, dynamic, and thermal allodynia, can be a significant problem for many patients with neuropathic pain. There is some evidence that opioids can be useful in treating dynamic allodynia, and the threshold for cold allodynia generally responds well in patients with peripheral neuropathic pain but not central neuropathic pain. There is no consistent evidence that opioids reduce the magnitude or threshold of static or heat allodynia. None of the studies selected for inclusion in the systematic review evaluated treatment durations in excess of 4 weeks. Evidence is stronger for oxycodone than for any of the other opioids. These experimental data are somewhat at odds with what might be expected from an examination of the neuroanatomical basis of opioid action. The majority of ORs in the dorsal horn of the spinal cord (predominately μ- and δ-receptors) are present on the presynaptic terminals of small C- and AD-fibres in the substantia gelatinosa. AD-fibres are thought to mediate static allodynias, whilst larger AB-fibres, which probably mediate dynamic allodynias, have a relative paucity of ORs.

12.4 **Central pain**

Although a number of high-quality short- or intermediate-term trials have included patients with neuropathic pain of both central and peripheral origin, it is difficult to draw firm conclusions concerning the opioid responsiveness of neuropathic pain of central origin. One study that is worth noting, however, compared a high- with a low-dose regimen of the potent μ-opioid levorphanol in 81 patients with centrally or peripherally generated neuropathic pain. All diagnostic subgroups of patients responded favourably, with pain intensity being reduced more with the high-strength regimen than with the low-strength regimen. There is some evidence, therefore, that centrally generated pain can respond to opioids, although opioid sensitivity may be reduced.

12.5 **Conclusion**

Opioids may reduce neuropathic pain intensity in the short to medium term, and there is evidence that opioids reduce some forms of evoked neuropathic pain. There are rationale theories as to why peripheral and central neuropathic pain may show reduced opioid sensitivity, although this has not been demonstrated in clinical practice.

The opioids with the strongest evidence for efficacy in neuropathic pain are morphine, oxycodone, and the weak μ-agonist tramadol. In the case of full μ-agonists, a meta-analysis has quantified the reduction in pain intensity due to opioids as being around 13 points on a 0–100 pain scale. One obvious, but important, question is whether this represents a clinically meaningful improvement in symptoms; another is whether conclusions regarding long-term treatment of neuropathic pain can be extrapolated from data obtained from trials lasting, at most, 10 weeks. Long-term longitudinal data are still required to answer these questions.

Key Reading

Arnér S and Myerson B (1988). Lack of analgesic effect of opioids on neuropathic and idiopathic forms of pain. *Pain*, **33**, 11–23.

Boureau F, Legallicier P, and Kabir-Ahmadi M (2003). Tramadol in post-herpetic neuralgia: a randomized, double-blind, placebo-controlled trial. *Pain*, **104**, 323–31.

Christoph T, De Vry J, and Tzschentke TM (2010). Tapentadol, but not morphine, selectively inhibits disease-related thermal hyperalgesia in a mouse model of diabetic neuropathic pain. *Neuroscience Letters*, **470**, 91–4.

Christoph T, De Vry J, Schiene K, Tallarida RJ, and Tzschentke TM (2011). Synergistic anti-hypersensitive effects of pregabalin and tapentadol in a rat model of neuropathic pain. *European Journal of Pharmacology*, **666**, 72–9.

Dellemijn P (1999). Are opioids effective in relieving neuropathic pain? *Pain*, **80**, 453–62.

Dickenson A and Suzuki R (2005). Opioids in neuropathic pain: clues from animal studies. *European Journal of Pain*, **9**, 113–16.

Eisenberg E, McNicol ED, and Carr DB (2005). Efficacy of μ-opioid agonists in the treatment of evoked neuropathic pain. Systemic review of randomized controlled trials. *European Journal of Pain*, **10**, 667–76.

Eisenberg E, McNicol E, and Carr DB (2006). Opioids for neuropathic pain (review). *Cochrane Database for Systematic Reviews*, CD006146.

Finnerup NB, Otto M, McQuay H, Jensen TS, and Sindrup SH (2005). Algorithm for neuropathic pain treatment: an evidence-based proposal. *Pain*, **118**, 289–305.

Finnerup NB, Sindrup SH, and Jensen TS (2010). The evidence for pharmacological treatment of neuropathic pain. *Pain*, **150**, 573–81.

Hollingshead J, Dühmke RM, and Cornblath DR (2006). Tramadol for neuropathic pain (review). *Cochrane Database for Systematic Reviews*, CD003726.

Kögel B, De Vry J, Tzschentke TM, and Christoph T (2011). The anti-nociceptive and anti-hyperalgesic effect of tapentadol is partially retained in OPRM1 (μ-opioid receptor) knock-out mice. *Neuroscience Letters*, **491**, 104–7.

Likar R and Sittl R (2005). Transdermal buprenorphine for treating nociceptive and neuropathic pain: four case studies. *Anesthesia & Analgesia*, **100**, 781–5.

Schwartz S, Etropolski M, Shapiro DY, Okamoto A, Lange R, Haeussler J et al. (2011). Safety and efficacy of tapentadol ER in patients with painful diabetic peripheral neuropathy: results of a randomized withdrawal, placebo-controlled trial. *Current Medical Research & Opinion*, **27**, 151–62.

Chapter 13

Practical aspects of prescribing

Key points

- There is no right or wrong type of patient suitable for opioid therapy.
- Opioids may play a partial role in the management of both nociceptive and neuropathic pain.
- The benefits and adverse effects of opioid treatment should be discussed with the patient and relevant others, and aims of therapy agreed and documented.
- Patients should undergo a trial of opioid therapy, with reasonable dose adjustment, active management of side effects, and monitoring of adverse effects and goals of treatment.
- There should be agreement between the prescriber and patient to stop opioid therapy if aims of treatment are not fulfilled within two or three dose adjustments.
- Harms of opioids are dose-related, and, in most circumstances, doses should not exceed 120 mg morphine equivalent per 24 hours.
- For most persistent pain conditions that are suitable for opioid therapy, sustained-release rather than immediate-release formulations are preferable.
- Clear allocation of responsibility for prescribing opioids in the long term should be agreed, including a plan for regular review of the patient to assess continuing utility of the opioid drug.
- Patients who fail to respond to one opioid drug may show a more favourable response with an alternative opioid.
- Tables describing relative potencies of opioids should serve as a guide only when switching a patient from one opioid to another.
- Caution should be exercised when switching a patient to or from methadone.
- The role of intrathecal opioid therapy in the management of persisting non-cancer pain needs further clarification.

13.1 Making a decision whether to prescribe opioids

In the … absence of scientific evidence, physicians are left to resort to their own attitudes and beliefs and the patients are left at the mercy of the physician's bias rather than the results of definite research.

Turk

13.1.1 **Influences on opioid prescribing**

The decision to prescribe strong opioid medication for a patient with long-term pain can be challenging for clinicians. Prescribers are subject to a number of influences, which, with individual interpretation, will shape beliefs about the effectiveness and safety of prescribing these drugs. These influences are discussed in the following sections.

Marketing of opioid products by the pharmaceutical industry
The influence of marketing on prescriber behaviour is well documented. There are many opioid products available to clinicians. Additionally, technical advances in the way that drugs can be delivered may have an intuitive pharmacological appeal, but robust data are lacking regarding the clinical benefit that a particular mode of administration may confer. Products can only be marketed for licensed indications, but diagnostic groups relating to chronic pain rarely have discrete boundaries, and inclusion of a particular clinical presentation within such a diagnostic group is open to flexible interpretation.

Guidelines and scientific research
A number of professionals in different countries have produced guidelines and recommendations regarding opioid prescribing. Many of these have been developed, with the aim of ensuring adequate pain relief to those who need it and, generally, are likely to increase rather than decrease the willingness to prescribe. Such guidelines are based on available evidence. Clinical trials of opioid therapy have seemed to support the use of opioids for a variety of pain conditions, and these have been evaluated by means of systematic review. However, well-documented trends towards more liberal prescribing of opioids have prompted professionals to re-examine the evidence and, in particular, to question the degree to which clinical trial data can be extrapolated to the long-term prescription of drugs.

Substance misuse concerns
Both patients and professionals misunderstand the terms 'addiction', 'dependence', 'tolerance', and 'problem drug use' (see Chapter 14). Beliefs about risk of addiction are a significant influence on doctors' willingness or otherwise to prescribe opioids. Again, guidelines and expert pronouncements are influencing current practice in a way likely to increase confidence in prescribing, even in patients with a history of substance misuse.

Availability of alternatives
Clinicians managing pain face the peculiar challenge that no class of drug works reliably in all patients and that, in those for whom benefit can be demonstrated, reduction in pain intensity may be moderate. This uncertainty of outcome may well influence the decision to prescribe an opioid drug. Increased understanding of potential adverse effects related to drugs in common use may limit therapeutic choice; for example, emerging data relating to gastrointestinal and cardiovascular safety of NSAIDs and cyclo-oxygenase-2 selective inhibitors are likely to act as a brake on indiscriminate prescribing of these drugs and of the over-the-counter use by patients. In the UK, the withdrawal of co-proxamol (a dextropropoxyphene/paracetamol combination drug) leaves a population of patients in pain in need of alternative pharmacotherapy.

Regulatory issues
The prescription of opioids is controlled within each country by a regulatory framework, and prescribers must act in accordance with the law. Mechanisms exist for monitoring the prescription of controlled drugs, and clinicians whose prescribing is thought

to be aberrant may face severe penalties. Fear of legislative scrutiny and the accompanying risk of professional opprobrium will inevitably discourage some pain therapists from prescribing opioids.

13.1.2 **Patient selection**

When faced with a difficult chronic pain problem, it may, or may not, be reassuring to know that there are no right answers. Some clinical situations may seem fairly straightforward; for example, an elderly patient with disabling arthritis, in whom medical comorbidity precludes joint replacement surgery, would probably be a good candidate for treatment with opioids if the benefits outweigh the adverse effects. Conversely, strong opioids would be inappropriate in the management of a young patient with simple mechanical low back pain. If opioids are to play a role in helping an individual patient, some general considerations regarding appropriate patient selection should apply.

Is this the right sort of patient?

Many clinicians will express concerns about the suitability of individual patients to receive opioids. These can rarely be substantiated by scientific facts, and prejudices are common. Unfortunately, the literature does not provide the answers. Received wisdom suggests that patients with comorbid psychiatric disorders or 'psychological problems' should not be prescribed opioids. One study suggests that patients with low back pain who have high levels of psychological distress may do less well when prescribed opioids than those who are less distressed, but the interpretation of this study has been debated. Individuals with mood disturbance, anxiety, and sleep problems may seek opioid prescriptions to attenuate these symptoms. Opioids should not be prescribed for this purpose for patients without pain. If a patient presents with disabling pain that is suitable for a trial of opioid therapy, comorbid disorders should not present a barrier to treatment but should be noted and treated appropriately. Similarly, although it is suggested that those who have a chaotic social background are not suitable for opioid treatment, the chaos should be explored and appropriate support enlisted to ensure safe implementation of whatever is the most appropriate therapy for the pain.

Patients with a past or current history of substance misuse, or who have a family member with such a history, give rise to some of the most challenging decisions regarding opioid treatment. These issues are discussed in more detail in Chapter 14.

13.1.3 **Prescribing for children and the elderly**

The uncertainty regarding the effects of opioids in the long term should prompt extreme caution when deciding on appropriate pharmacological therapy for children with persistent pain. Adequate analgesia should not be denied to children with painful, often progressive, debilitating conditions, but decisions to prescribe opioids should be carried out by an experienced multi-professional childrens' pain management team, in close collaboration with the child's family doctor.

There are few good-quality studies in the literature to guide the therapist regarding prescription of opioids for the elderly. Clinical trials of opioid efficacy tend to exclude older patients and those with comorbid disease. Pharmacokinetic studies relating to opioids in the elderly usually relate to single or short-term administration of drugs. Effects of ageing relevant to the prescription of opioids include:

- Increased incidence of adverse effects of drugs in the elderly
- Increased frequency of drug interactions and likelihood of polypharmacy

- Increased medical comorbidity
- Pharmacokinetic considerations, including altered volume of distribution of opioid drugs and potentially impaired metabolism and excretion
- Altered pharmacodynamics of opioid drugs related to influences on neurotransmitter release and receptor population.

The elderly person in pain can safely be prescribed opioids, but starting doses should be cautious. Older patients should be reviewed frequently to assess efficacy and side effects of opioids, and to allow dose adjustment until useful analgesia is achieved.

Does the patient have the right sort of pain?
The distinction between nociceptive and neuropathic pain is probably not important when evaluating a patient for opioid treatment, as both types of pain are opioid-responsive to a degree and many patients present a mixed picture. Central pain syndromes are notoriously refractory to treatment, but limited trial data suggest that a trial of opioids in patients with central pain may be worthwhile.

There are some pain syndromes for which the efficacy of a number of interventions has been evaluated and in which opioids have less evidence to support their use than other management approaches. These include simple mechanical back pain and fibromyalgia (in the latter, there is poor evidence for efficacy of strong opioids other than tramadol for which there is weak evidence.); this does not mean that use of strong opioids in such conditions is contraindicated, but good practice would dictate that interventions that are more likely to succeed should be properly pursued initially. The management of so-called idiopathic chronic pain syndromes, i.e. conditions where the aetiology of symptoms cannot be explained, is controversial, and the use of long-term opioids for pain relief in these circumstances is usually agreed to be inappropriate. These challenging cases exemplify the importance of comprehensive assessment by an experienced multidisciplinary pain management team.

Is this the best time to prescribe opioids?
Opioids have traditionally been considered a treatment of last resort when all other therapies have failed. Certainly concerns about the safety and efficacy of opioids when prescribed in the long term should prompt caution when prescribing, but therapies offered earlier in the care pathway should have a reasonable evidence base when applied to the condition being treated; for example, a patient with neuropathic pain might reasonably be started on amitriptyline or an anti-epileptic medication as first-line treatment. The utility of non-pharmacological interventions, including advice regarding activity, paced increase in exercise, and behavioural interventions as well as physical modalities such as TENS, should be explored and applied where appropriate before considering opioid therapy. Opioids should rarely be prescribed in isolation; it is more usual to deliver opioid therapy in parallel with other partially successful interventions and in the wider context of a multidisciplinary approach to pain management.

The patient with persistent pain who presents to acute medical services, often in secondary care, merits special consideration as do individuals in hospital with pain, which persists despite surgery intended to alleviate symptoms. An acute hospital ward provides a poor context in which to evaluate the complexities of a chronic pain problem and make a rational treatment plan. Pressures to minimize hospital bed occupancy may lead clinical teams to look for quick solutions, and, in this regard, strategies of proven utility in the management of acute pain, including the prescription of opioids, are appealing. Treatment may be started without considered discussion with the patient regarding the benefits and burdens of opioid therapy in the long term, and without an agreed treatment plan that identifies goals of therapy and indicates how these might be achieved. Inappropriate prescribing, although sometimes providing short-term answers, can be counterproductive and can result in an unhelpful dependency on acute medical services. Clinical teams should be encouraged to engage the help of chronic pain professionals in formulating a realistic discharge plan at an early stage in any such admission.

13.2 **Starting a patient on strong opioid medication**

Opioids should be prescribed for chronic pain as part of an overall rehabilitation plan, which addresses not only relevant medical interventions but also includes strategies for managing the physical, emotional, social, and vocational needs of the patient with persistent pain. It is important that the patient recognizes that opioid therapy is part of this larger plan.

The plan should be discussed with the patient and his or her relatives or carers. Goals of therapy should be discussed, and a reasonable time by which they should be achieved should be agreed.

Before prescribing opioids in the long term, it is important that a closely monitored trial of opioid therapy is carried out. Testing of responsiveness to intravenously administered opioids has been advocated as a means of avoiding the need for a prolonged trial of oral opioid therapy. Such testing has a useful negative predictive power but may give little useful information regarding the efficacy of opioids in the long term or the acceptability, or otherwise, of adverse effects. A supervised trial of oral or transdermal therapy over a period of weeks or months gives a more useful indication of the likely response to long-term opioid therapy.

13.2.1 **The opioid trial**

The primary purpose of prescribing opioids is to reduce the intensity of pain as a means of supporting rehabilitation. Complete relief of symptoms is rarely achievable; an acceptable balance between useful reduction in pain intensity and side effects is the goal. This balance will need regular evaluation. Improvements in physical, psychological, and social function are important secondary outcomes of opioid treatment and should be monitored at each assessment.

The duration of the opioid trial should be agreed with the patient. The trial should be carried out at a time when the patient and therapist are able to meet together regularly to assess progress and monitor problems. The frequency of patient review during the trial may be constrained by the availability of consulting time but, where possible, should be, at least, monthly, and the patient must be given clear instructions regarding sources of help regarding his or her therapy between visits. It is usual for the therapist initiating the opioid trial to issue repeat prescriptions during the trial and to evaluate the patient, but it is important that other health care professionals responsible for the patient are informed of the treatment plan. The patient should be started on a low dose of opioid. Upward adjustments of the dose can be made either by the patient, with clear instructions from the prescriber, or by the therapist at each review. It is usual to expect two or three such adjustments of the dose during the trial of therapy. If the patient does not achieve useful relief of symptoms, or develops intolerable side effects after reasonable dose adjustment, the opioid trial should be deemed unsuccessful.

Potential adverse effects of opioids should be discussed. Common side effects, such as sedation, sweating, nausea, mood change, and constipation, should be emphasized. It is helpful to explain that tolerance to some side effects, particularly sedation and nausea, may occur within a few days of starting treatment and that, where possible, these side effects will be actively managed. The effects of opioids on skills relevant to driving should be discussed (see Chapter 7). Although research suggests that patients on stable doses of opioids are generally safe to drive, patients should be advised to avoid driving when first taking opioids and following upward adjustment in dose. The patient must evaluate critically his or her fitness to drive safely on each occasion when they wish to do so. Patients should also be advised to discuss their medication with the appropriate vehicle licensing authorities and their motor insurance company.

The patient should be reminded of the importance of looking after the opioid prescription carefully and of the need to store controlled drugs safely. It should be emphasized that the law proscribes the use of controlled drugs by anyone other than the intended recipient.

Long-term adverse effects of opioids, including hormonal dysfunction and immunosuppression, should be discussed. It is also useful to discuss the definitions of dependence, tolerance, and addiction in relation to the use of opioids for pain control, and it may be useful to highlight symptoms and signs of intoxication and withdrawal from opioids to the patient and his or her carers. The patient should be questioned regarding current or past history of substance misuse, and it is helpful to discuss sensitively whether other members of the patient's family or household have substance misuse problems.

It is helpful to support the clinical discussion with provision of written or taped information. Where possible, a patient should be given time to consider the implications of a trial of opioid treatment and the use of these drugs in the longer term. They may wish to discuss treatment with family members or other health care professionals before reaching a decision.

Discussions regarding opioid therapy should be documented in the medical records. Some centres use a more formalized opioid contract. The material included in the contract varies, although the conditions under which opioid therapy will be discontinued are usually outlined. The efficacy of opioid contracts has not been validated, and their legal status is questionable.

13.2.2 **Choice of drug**

There is little in the literature to support the use of any specific opioid drug for a given indication. It is usual, therefore, to start therapy with modified-release morphine, although there is a rationale for changing drugs in an individual patient if the first-line drug fails to provide useful attenuation of symptoms or if it is associated with unacceptable side effects.

For pain associated with cancer, the use of modified-release analgesic preparations to provide background analgesia, with rapidly acting formulations for breakthrough pain, is recommended. In the case of persistent non-cancer pain, it is usual to use sustained-release preparations only, although a systematic review of the literature does not support the idea that sustained-release preparations provide more effective

Table 13.1 Long-acting opioids	
Pharmaceutically long-acting opioids	Inherently (pharmacologically) long-acting opioids
Buprenorphine transdermal	
Dihydrocodeine modified release	
Fentanyl transdermal	Levorphanol
Hydromorphone modified release	Methadone
Morphine modified release	
Oxycodone modified release	
Tapentadol modified release	

Adapted from Jackson KC (2005), Chapter 3, 'Opioid pharmacokinetics', in MP Davis, P Glare, and J Hardy (eds.). *Opioids in Cancer Pain*, p. 43, by permission of Oxford University Press.

analgesia. Of the commonly used opioids, methadone and levorphanol (not currently available in the UK) are intrinsically long-acting. Long-acting formulations are now available for other opioid drugs (see Table 13.1). Generally, the use of regular, time-contingent medication is considered a better support to a rehabilitative plan, compared to the irregular use of medication in response to pain. Patients need to understand that the use of sustained-release preparations will result in periods when pain is less well controlled. For most patients, pain intensity fluctuates, so an opioid dose which provides relief of the most severe symptoms could result in considerable, and potentially dangerous, overmedication during periods when the pain is less severe.

Injectable preparations are rarely, if ever, justified in the management of non-cancer pain syndromes.

Although the use of sustained-release preparations, as described, is advisable for most persistent pain syndromes, the individual presentation should be considered. Patients who describe very intermittent spontaneous pain, who have pain only at certain times of day, or who have infrequent incident pain (where pain is provoked by a particular activity) may be considered for an opioid regimen that includes (or is based solely upon) immediate-release preparations. A recent study has suggested that for selected patients, the use of immediate-release, or immediate in combination with controlled-release, medication may result in an overall reduction in daily opioid load and in perceived problems associated with treatment. Such regimens need close monitoring and appropriate adjustment, and specialist advice is recommended.

Acute visceral pain may be augmented by smooth muscle spasm in the affected organ, and an example of this is the pain of biliary colic. All opioids cause an increase in biliary pressure, but studies performed in the 1960s indicated that pethidine caused less intense biliary spasm than morphine. This is thought to be due to the additional mild alpha-blockade and anticholinergic effects that are exhibited by pethidine, and this led to it being the drug of choice to treat the pain of biliary or renal colic. It is now believed that, in equianalgesic doses, pethidine does not confer an advantage over other opioids when treating visceral pain, and the high lipid solubility of pethidine and the rapid onset/offset of effect may predispose to problem drug use. Additionally, its active metabolite (norpethidine) may give rise to serious CNS side effects (see Section 2.5.1, Chapter 2).

13.2.3 **Opioid dose**

Effectiveness data suggest that doses of opioid averaging 120 mg morphine equivalent/ day may have a role in the management of persistent pain. In practice, the doses of opioids used often far exceed those known to be safe and effective in the context of clinical trials. There is robust evidence to show that harms of treatment are dose-related. In most cases, opioids should be titrated to a maximum of 120 mg morphine equivalent per 24 hours for patients who are not currently using opioids; if there is no demonstrable benefit at this dose, further upward dose adjustment is unlikely to be helpful, and the drug should be tapered and stopped. If opioid cessation is not possible, current recommendations suggest such patients should be reviewed by a specialist.

This does not mean that opioid doses equivalent to greater than 120 mg morphine/24 hours should never be used; if such doses are providing both useful relief of symptoms and improvement in function, it is reasonable to continue the high-dose prescription, but continued utility should be assessed frequently.

13.3 **Prescribing opioids in the long term**

A trial of opioid therapy can be considered successful if the patient reports an unequivocal useful reduction in the intrusiveness of his or her pain, in the absence of troubling side effects. This reduction in pain should be accompanied by the achievement of previously agreed functional goals.

13.3.1 **Stopping opioid therapy**

The plan for prescription of opioids in the long term should be agreed with the patient, and this should include a discussion of whether a trial of cessation of therapy should take place. In certain circumstances, e.g. when opioids are being prescribed for symptomatic relief whilst a patient is awaiting potentially pain-relieving surgery (e.g. joint replacement), it is clear that a tapering of opioid dose should take place when the patient is recovered from his or her operation. Long-term opioids should be used properly to support a rehabilitative plan, and a cautious exploration of the continued utility of the drugs is reasonable when the patient feels that he or she has achieved a sustained improvement in function. When opioids are being prescribed for painful conditions that have an unfavourable natural history, e.g. central neuropathic pain syndromes, the duration of therapy is less clear-cut. Patients should be reminded of the long-term adverse effects of the drugs and the importance of only taking drugs (of any class) that confer substantial benefit.

Other situations in which the continuation of opioid treatment should be evaluated carefully include the emergence of a substance misuse problem (see Chapter 14) or subsequent failure to achieve useful pain control despite reasonable adjustment in dose. The clinical syndrome of opioid-induced hyperalgesia is now well described, although the frequency with which this occurs in clinical practice is unclear (see Chapter 8). If the diagnosis is suspected, the patient will need management by a specialist team, and this may be effected most easily in an inpatient setting.

Cessation of opioid therapy requires cooperation between the patient and health care professionals. The dose should be tapered gradually to allow the patient to evaluate the effect of dose reduction on pain and function, and to minimize symptoms of opioid withdrawal. Patients should be given sufficient information to enable them to recognize symptoms of withdrawal. Resolution of withdrawal symptoms may occur by reducing the rate of dose reduction, but, occasionally, such symptoms may need active pharmacological management.

13.3.2 Responsibility for prescribing

If a patient is to be treated with long-term opioid therapy, the responsibility for providing prescriptions should be agreed. For most patients, it is most sensible for prescriptions to be supplied by their primary care practitioner. The primary care practitioner should have the continued support of a specialist pain management team if needed, particularly if the opioid therapy has been initiated by the specialist team. Where possible, patients should receive prescriptions from one source only, but provision should be made to ensure continuity of prescription when the prescriber is unavailable. If a clinician who is not the patient's regular prescriber is asked for a prescription, he or she should ascertain why the prescription cannot come from the usual source and should alert the patient's regular prescriber that a prescription has been issued.

13.3.3 Frequency of review

The frequency with which the patient receiving long-term opioids is followed up will depend on the individual clinical situation. For patients with a stable condition, who achieve useful pain relief from a moderate dose of opioids and who do not appear to develop tolerance to the drug, a 6-monthly review may be adequate. Patients who need high doses of opioid, and, in particular, those using immediate-release preparations as part of their regimen, will need much more frequent assessment. These more complex patients will need the continuing input of a specialist pain management team. Reluctance by the patient to attend for follow-up and discuss his or her opioid regimen should prompt urgent re-evaluation of the continuing benefits of therapy.

13.4 Changing opioid regimen

13.4.1 Clinical background

The published literature does not indicate superiority of efficacy of any one opioid preparation over another if given in equianalgesic doses. Similarly, there are no large trials comparing opioids, which provide evidence of benefit in terms of adverse effects. However, the long-observed inter-individual variability in analgesic response to morphine and other opioids and the varied susceptibility to side effects has given impetus to the practice of opioid switching. This pragmatic approach assumes that a patient who fails to derive analgesia from their initial opioid regimen or who develops intolerable side effects can successfully be prescribed an alternative opioid to improve the balance of benefits and adverse effects. Opioid switching (sometimes described as opioid rotation, which strictly implies return to the original opioid regimen) is well described in the cancer pain literature and is increasingly incorporated into practice when prescribing opioids for non-cancer pain. Prospective studies of opioid switching (many of which were uncontrolled) have been systematically reviewed and confirm that the practice appears to be effective, both in terms of improving analgesic efficacy and of minimizing opioid-induced adverse effects. However, the evidence base for opioid switching is weakened by a lack of data from randomized controlled trials and the inconsistency of the published material regarding diagnostic category, comorbidity, and route of administration.

13.4.2 **Scientific rationale**

There are many influences which determine a patient's response to a drug. Some of these, including expectations, mood, pain severity, and the context of the therapy, might be expected to be comparable across a number of drugs of the same class. There are a number of reasons why an individual patient may respond to one opioid more favourably than another. These include differences in pharmacokinetics and pharmacodynamics of opioid drugs between patients. The genetic basis of this variability has now been well researched and reported, and includes:

- Variability in OR population and density
- Polymorphism in genes coding for the drug transporter
- Polymorphism in the μ-OR gene
- Influences on genetic variation in enzymes involved in opioid metabolism
- Genetic differences in other neurochemical systems that influence opioid response (NMDA, dopamine, serotonin).

13.4.3 **Clinical implications**

Safe practice in opioid switching must be underpinned by the knowledge of the relative potencies of the available opioid preparations when given by different routes (see Appendix 2). However, such conversion tables, which are usually derived from single-dose studies, must be interpreted with caution. Experimental data demonstrate that conversion ratios vary considerably between individuals (for the reasons outlined in Section 13.4 Changing opioid regimen), and it is unsurprising that many quite disparate conversion tables are available in the published literature. It is important to take an individualized approach to opioid switching, and relative potencies should act as a guide only. The starting dose of the new drug will depend on whether the switch is being made because of inefficacy of the current regimen or because of current side effects. A relative reduction in opioid dose is often observed when changing from one preparation to another as a result of incomplete cross-tolerance, and it is reasonable to make a conservative conversion initially, with close monitoring and upward titration of the new drug as appropriate. Additionally, conversion ratios demonstrate directionality; it is, therefore, unsafe to assume that a further switch to the original drug can be effected simply by prescribing the former dose, as the response to a drug depends on the preceding opioid regimen.

13.4.4 **Conversion to methadone**

Much of the literature on opioid switching relates to the introduction of methadone to replace an existing opioid regimen. Methadone has a number of pharmacologic properties, which confer advantages in the management of persistent pain but also necessitate caution when prescribing the drug.

Methadone has high affinity for both μ- and δ-ORs. It has been demonstrated in animals to have activity at the NMDA receptor, which gives the drug intuitive appeal in the management of neuropathic pain and in cases of apparent tolerance to alternative opioid preparations. The drug has high and relatively consistent oral bioavailability (around 85%) and is rapidly absorbed. It is extensively metabolized in the liver to inactive metabolites. Methadone has a large volume of distribution, and its slow release from extravascular sites give the drug its long and unpredictable half-life, which, although an advantage in the management of persisting symptoms as it allows infrequent dosing, brings a significant associated risk of accumulation and delayed toxicity. Steady-state and maximal analgesia may take five days or more to achieve. Conversion to methadone, therefore, requires careful titration and, particularly, close observation. Conversion can most easily be achieved in an inpatient setting. Particular care is needed when switching to methadone from high doses of alternative opioids (as conversion ratios vary substantially, depending on the starting dose of the original opioid, and may change during therapy) and when methadone is taken with other sedative drugs, including benzodiazepines, antidepressants, and alcohol.

A number of different strategies for establishing a patient on methadone have been described. The authors use an adapted version of the regimen described by Morley and Makin (see Appendix 3).

The increasing popularity of methadone as an analgesic will inevitably lead to more frequent switching from methadone to an alternative drug. Conversion ratios for substituting methadone with other opioids are not well described and indeed may vary considerably from patient to patient. Conversion from methadone may be accompanied by a marked increase in pain, refractory to escalation of the dose of the new drug.

13.5 **Intrathecal opioid therapy**

The identification of ORs in the spinal cord and subsequent demonstration in animals of potent analgesia following intrathecal injection of opioids provided a sound rationale for the use of spinally administered opioids to treat pain in man. Techniques for delivering opioids spinally in the short term for the management of post-operative and other acute pains are now well established. Similarly, the use of intrathecal opioids to improve efficacy and minimize side effects of therapy in patients at the end of life is now an established technique in specialized settings. The long-term use of opioids delivered intrathecally for persistent non-cancer pain is more controversial. The efficacy of the technique is not well proven, and concerns exist regarding adverse effects, particularly relating to the endocrine system (see further below in this section) and opioid tolerance. There is poor agreement regarding the type of pain problem that is most likely to be helped by this treatment.

Delivery of opioids over prolonged periods for patients with non-cancer-related pain is usually by means of a fully implanted system, with an intrathecal catheter connected to a programmable pump that delivers the drug to the cerebrospinal fluid. These systems are expensive, and device-related problems may occur in up to 40% of patients. The pump requires regular refill with the drug by a health care professional.

There are many retrospective, and some prospective, uncontrolled studies in the literature, which demonstrate that, over the medium term, patients remain satisfied with the therapy and continue to report a reduction in pain. Return to work, however, is a rarely achieved goal, possibly because patients selected for treatment are those with the most severe and unremitting symptoms that have generally been refractory to other pain therapies. One prospective controlled study compared patients meeting local criteria for intrathecal therapy who exhibited substantial relief of pain following a trial of treatment and who progressed to long-term therapy with those who did not get relief during the trial or did not wish to go ahead with the implantation of a programmable pump. New referrals to the unit, who were managed with interventions other than intrathecal therapy, comprised a second control group. Outcomes were evaluated (over a period of 3 years) by means of validated instruments for the measurement of pain, mood, and function. The study demonstrated improvements in pain, mood, and function for the implanted group (many of whom received additional intrathecal drugs such as clonidine, local anaesthetic, or baclofen) compared to those who had failed the intrathecal opioid trial but less improvement in these domains compared to the new referrals to the unit.

The endocrine effects of intrathecal opioid treatment have been characterized in some detail. Therapy is associated with hypothalamic/pituitary/gonadal suppression, resulting in decreased libido in both sexes, with erectile dysfunction in men and menstrual disturbances in women. Hypogonadism may occur, and supplemental endocrine treatment may be necessary.

Intrathecal opioid therapy remains a popular therapy in some centres. There is a pressing need for further research regarding the balance of benefits to patients and risks of long-term health problems.

Key Reading

Abs R, Verhelst J, Maeyaert J, Van Buyten JP, Opsomer F, Adriaensen H et al. (2000). Endocrine consequences of long-term intrathecal administration of opioids. *Journal of Clinical Endocrinology and Metabolism*, **85**, 2215–22.

British Pain Society (2008). Intrathecal drug delivery for the management of pain and spasticity in adults: recommendations for best clinical practice. Available from: http://www.britishpainsociety.org/book_ittd_main.pdf [Accessed November 26, 2012].

British Pain Society (2010). Opioids for persistent pain: good practice. Available from: http://www.britishpainsociety.org/pub_professional.htm#opioids [Accessed November 26, 2012].

British Pain Society (2010). Opioid medicines for persistent pain: information for patients. Available from: http://www.britishpainsociety.org/book_opioid_patient.pdf [Accessed November 26, 2012].

Chou R, Clark E, and Helfand M (2003). Comparative efficacy and safety of long-acting oral opioids for chronic non-cancer pain: a systematic review. *Journal of Pain and Symptom Management*, **26**, 1026–48.

Chou R, Fanciullo GJ, Fine PG, Adler JA, Ballantyne JC, Davies P et al. American Pain Society-American Academy of Pain Medicine Opioids Guidelines Panel (2009). Clinical guidelines for the use of chronic opioid therapy in chronic non-cancer pain. *Journal of Pain*, **10**, 113–30.

De C Williams AC (2005). Psychological distress and opioid efficacy: more questions than answers. *Pain*, **117**, 245–6.

Eisenberg E, McNicol E, and Carr DB (2006). Opioids for neuropathic pain. *Cochrane Database of Systematic Reviews*, CD006146.

Fishman SM and Kreis PG (2002). The opioid contract. *Clinical Journal of Pain*, **18**, S70–5.

Gouke CR (2001). Australian management strategies for oral opioid use in non-malignant pain. *European Journal of Pain*, **5**, 99–101.

Gustorff B (2005). Intravenous opioid testing in patients with chronic non-cancer pain. *European Journal of Pain*, **9**, 123–5.

Haddox JD, Joranson DE, Angarola RT, Brady A, Carr DB, Blonsky ER et al. (1997). The use of opioids for the treatment of chronic pain. A consensus statement from the American Academy of Pain Medicine and the American Pain Society. *Clinical Journal of Pain*, **13**, 6–8.

Hutchinson K, Moreland ME, de C Williams AC, Weinman J, and Horne R (2007). Exploring beliefs and practice of opioid prescribing for persistent non-cancer pain by general practitioners. *European Journal of Pain*, **11**, 93–8.

Moryl N, Santiago-Palma J, Komick C, Derby S, Fischberg D, Payne R et al. (2002). Pitfalls of opioid rotation: substituting another opioid for methadone in patients with cancer pain. *Pain*, **96**, 325–8.

Nicholson AB (2004). Methadone for cancer pain. *Cochrane Database of Systematic Reviews*, CD003971.

Portenoy RK and Savage SR (1997). Clinical realities and economic considerations: special therapeutic issues in intrathecal therapy—tolerance and addiction. *Journal of Pain and Symptom Management*, **14**, S27–35.

Quigley C (2004). Opioid switching to improve pain relief and drug tolerability. *Cochrane Database of Systematic Reviews*, CD004847.

Ross JR, Riley J, Quigley C, and Welsh KI (2006). Clinical pharmacology and pharmacotherapy of opioid switching in cancer patients. *Oncologist*, **11**, 765–73.

Stamer UM, Bayerer B, and Stuber F (2005). Genetics and variability in opioid response. *European Journal of Pain*, **9**, 101–4.

Stannard CF (2011). Opioids for chronic pain: promise and pitfalls. *Current Opinion in Supportive and Palliative Care*, **5**, 150–7.

Thimineur MA, Kravitz E, and Vodapally MS (2004). Intrathecal opioid treatment for chronic non-malignant pain; a 3-year prospective study. *Pain*, **109**, 242–9.

Turk DC, Brody MC, and Okifuji EA (1994). Physicians' attitudes and practices regarding the long-term prescribing of opioids for non-cancer pain. *Pain*, **59**, 201–8.

Twycross R, Wilcock A, Charlesworth S, and Dickman A (1998). *Palliative care formulary*. 2nd edn. Radcliffe Medical Press, Oxford.

Von Korff M, Merrill JO, Rutter CM, Sullivan M, Campbell CI, and Weisner C (2011). Time-scheduled vs pain-contingent opioid dosing in chronic opioid therapy. *Pain*, **152**, 1256–62.

Wasan A, Davar G, and Jamison R (2005). The association between negative affect and opioid analgesia in patients with discogenic low back pain. *Pain*, **117**, 450–61.

Washington State Agency Medical Directors Group (2010). Interagency guideline on opioid dosing for chronic non-cancer pain: an educational aid to improve care and safety with opioid therapy. Available from: http://www.agencymeddirectors.wa.gov/Files/OpioidGdline.pdf [Accessed November 26, 2012].

Wilder-Smith OHG (2005). Opioid use in the elderly. *European Journal of Pain*, **9**, 137–40.

Chapter 14

Opioids and addiction

Key points

- The utility of existing definitions of addiction, dependence, and tolerance when prescribing opioids for pain are debated.
- The syndrome of addiction is characterized by changes in the brain's motivational and reward circuitry.
- The prevalence of addiction to prescribed opioids has been variably reported.
- Prediction of the risk of addiction to prescribed opioids is difficult.
- Patients in pain with a past or current history of substance misuse can be managed with opioid drugs if given appropriate support and monitoring.
- Collaboration between the patient and all health care professionals with whom they are involved underpins safe prescribing of opioids.

14.1 Introduction

Persistent pain is hard to treat, and many, if not all, of the therapies available help a small proportion of patients, and efficacy is modest at best. In practice, patients with pain will be offered a number of therapeutic interventions, including different classes of analgesic drugs such as strong opioids. However, considerable speculation remains regarding the safety of opioids in the longer term. In particular, the concerns of clinicians regarding the propensity of these drugs to cause problems of tolerance, dependence, and addiction, which have, for many years, acted as a barrier to the prescribing of opioids, remain largely unanswered. These concerns become more prominent when prescribing opioid analgesic drugs for patients in pain who have a past or current history of substance misuse.

14.2 Substance misuse: size of the problem

Dependence on psychoactive substances is common throughout the world. Data from the UK suggest that in 2010/11, 8.8% of adults in England and Wales had used an illicit drug in the previous year, with cannabis being the most popular drug (6.8% adults). The highest drug use was seen in 16–19 year olds (28%). The use of drugs increases in those who drink alcohol frequently. Data from other developed countries suggest a problem of similar scale. The vast majority of these individuals do not receive treatment for substance misuse.

The problem of substance misuse imposes significant burdens on the individual and on society. The individual consequences have been classified into four groups:

1. Chronic health effects (cirrhosis, HIV, hepatitis)
2. Acute health effects (overdose, injury whilst intoxicated)
3. Acute social problems (arrest, disruption of relationship)
4. Chronic social problems (disruption of family role, effect on employment, low income).

The societal burden of substance misuse includes health care costs of both acute and chronic illness, costs in relation to criminal behaviour, and the burden of poor productivity and absenteeism from work in addition to long-term unemployment.

14.3 **Substance misuse: definitions**

Confusion regarding both the definition of terms relating to the use of psychoactive substances and diagnostic criteria for addiction has confounded the evaluation of problem drug use in relation to the treatment of pain. Existing diagnostic criteria relating to substance dependence, whilst of considerable applicability in the field of addiction medicine, serve to cause confusion when prescribing opioids for pain relief and have acted both as a barrier to appropriate prescribing of these drugs and as a source of concern to patients and their carers. The term 'substance dependence' itself, whilst widely accepted as being preferable to the term 'addiction', has a specific and quite distinct meaning when describing phenomena associated with prescribed drugs for pain relief (see further below in this section). The most commonly used criteria for substance dependence are the International Classification of Diseases, tenth revision (ICD-10) (see Box 14.1), and the fourth edition of the Diagnostic and Statistical Manual (DSM-IV) of the American Psychiatric Association (for further information see the website of the American Psychiatric Association, http://www.psychiatry.org/practice/dsm).

These criteria include the phenomena of tolerance and withdrawal as indicators of substance dependence, which, in the context of pain management, might result in over-diagnosis of an addiction syndrome. The criteria highlight the fact that addiction does not represent a single phenomenon but rather a pattern of substance misuse observed over time. A set of diagnostic criteria, applicable to individuals being prescribed opioids for pain, were developed by Portenoy (see Box 14.2).

> ### Box 14.1 Criteria for substance dependence in ICD-10
>
> Three or more of the following must have been experienced or exhibited together at some time during the previous year:
>
> 1. A strong desire or sense of compulsion to take the substance
> 2. Difficulties in controlling substance-taking behaviour, in terms of its onset, termination, or levels of use
> 3. A physiological withdrawal state when substance use has ceased or been reduced, as evidenced by: the characteristic withdrawal syndrome for the substance, or use of the same (or a closely related) substance with the intention of relieving or avoiding withdrawal symptoms
> 4. Evidence of tolerance such that increased doses of the psychoactive substance are required in order to achieve effects originally produced by lower doses
> 5. Progressive neglect of alternative pleasures or interests because of psychoactive substance use, increased amount of time necessary to obtain or take the substance or to recover from its effects
> 6. Persisting with substance use despite clear evidence of overtly harmful consequences such as harm to the liver through excessive drinking, depressive mood states consequent to heavy substance use, or drug-related impairment of cognitive functioning. Efforts should be made to determine that the user was actually, or could be expected to be, aware of the nature and extent of the harm.

WHO (1992). The ICD-10 classification of mental and behavioural disorders: clinical descriptions and diagnostic guidelines. World Health Organization, Geneva.

The confusion regarding the terminology for patients in pain using opioids medicinally had been resolved by the production of a clarifying consensus statement from the American Academy of Pain Medicine (AAPM), the American Pain Society (APS), and the American Society for Addiction Medicine (ASAM) (see Box 11.4). These definitions distinguished between expected sequelae of opioid therapy, including physical dependence and tolerance, and the more biologically and behaviourally complex syndrome of addiction.

Box 14.2 Criteria for diagnosing addiction in the context of patients taking opioids for chronic pain

Addiction is a psychological and behavioural syndrome characterized by:

1. An intense desire for the drug and overwhelming concern about its continued availability (psychological dependence)
2. Evidence of compulsive drug use, characterized by, for example:
   a) Unsanctioned dose escalation
   b) Continued dosing despite significant side effects
   c) Use of drugs to treat symptoms not targeted by therapy, or
   d) Unapproved use during periods of no symptoms, and/or
3. Evidence of one or more of a group of associated behaviours, including:
   a) Manipulation of the treating physician or medical system for the purpose of obtaining additional drug (e.g. by altering prescriptions)
   b) Acquisition of drugs from other medical sources or from non-medical sources
   c) Drug hoarding or sales
   d) Unapproved use of other drugs (particularly alcohol or other sedatives/hypnotics) during opioid therapy.

Portenoy, R.K. (1990). Chronic opioid therapy in non-malignant pain. J Pain Symptom Manage. 5, S46–62.

The definitions identified three key components of addiction:

- Impaired control over drug use
- Craving or compulsion regarding drug use
- Continued use despite harm.

Problems of evaluating addiction in the presence of unrelieved pain, which may itself be accompanied by apparently aberrant patterns of drug use, were highlighted in the AAPM/APS/ASAM consensus statement. The term 'pseudoaddiction' was coined to a pattern of behaviours, such as drug hoarding and attempts to procure extra supplies (as well as more worrisome behaviours, including illicit drug use and deception), that might usually be indicative of an addiction problem but which resolve on adequate treatment of pain.

Withdrawal is a syndrome observed following the cessation, or rapid dose reduction, of a drug or following the administration of a drug-specific antagonist. It is sometimes divided into psychological phenomena, such as craving, anhedonia and agitation, and physical phenomena such as diarrhoea or tachycardia. Withdrawal is well recognized in relation to the use of opioids but occurs with other drug classes, including alpha-2 agonists and corticosteroids.

What is now increasingly recognized is that individuals with pain receiving opioids may present with problems that are as complex to manage as those of addiction, and recognizing that addiction may complicate pain management is an important component of identifying patient needs and providing appropriate support. The drivers to continued opioid use may be numerous, and simple detoxification is unlikely to help in the absence of support for managing not only pain and comorbid mental health diagnoses but also social and vocational problems. Patients with addiction to, and problematic use of, opioids present complex challenges and need to be managed by multidisciplinary teams with skills in pain management and in addiction medicine.

Addiction
Addiction is a primary chronic neurobiologic disease, with genetic, psychosocial, and environmental factors influencing its development and manifestations. It is characterized by behaviours that include one or more of the following: impaired control over drug use, compulsive use, continued use despite harm, and craving.

Physical dependence
Physical dependence is a state of adaptation that is manifested by a drug class-specific withdrawal syndrome that can be produced by abrupt cessation, rapid dose reduction, decreasing blood level of the drug, and/or administration of an antagonist.

Tolerance
Tolerance is a state of adaptation in which exposure to a drug induces changes that result in a diminution of one or more of the drug effects over time.

American Academy of Pain Medicine, the American Pain Society, and the American Society of Addiction Medicine. Consensus statement: definitions related to the use of opioids for the treatment of pain. Available from: http:// www.ampainsoc.org/advocacy/opioids2.htm. Accessed May 2007.

14.4 **Neurobiology of addiction**

Addiction is a chronic relapsing brain disorder in which repeated exposure to certain substances induces change in motivational and reward systems of the brain. The widely held idea that the addicted individual has choice over his or her own behaviour in regard to drug taking has been refuted robustly by a massive increase in understanding of the neurobiological basis of the observed shift from the voluntary control over drug taking to the behaviourally complex syndrome of addiction. It is now known, from animal models and from functional imaging in man, that repeated exposure to a drug leads to a reorganization of neural circuitry as a result of:

• An increase in neurotransmitter release

• A change in receptor population

• A change in receptor signalling

• A change in ion channels

• Alterations in synaptic structure.

Systems that are usually involved in directing behaviour towards stimuli critical for survival are 'hijacked' such that drug-seeking behaviours become unavoidably the most compelling priority for the addicted individual.

Exposure to psychoactive substances does not produce a syndrome of addiction in all individuals. The likelihood of developing addiction and the manifestations of the disorder are influenced by genetic, psychologic, environmental, and social factors.

Substances that are misused generate pleasurable reward when ingested. The likelihood of an individual choosing to use psychoactive substances initially will be determined by his or her biological make-up as well as a number of environmental and social influences. These influences, in addition to the nature of the reward induced, also shape the propensity of the individual to repeated drug exposure. Neither can the complex behaviours associated with the syndrome of addiction be explained by a desire to induce reward alone nor can the avoidance of withdrawal symptoms be sufficient explanation for the phenomenon.

Important components of the reward circuitry of the brain include:

- The midbrain ventral tegmental area (VTA)
- The basal forebrain, including the nucleus accumbens
- The frontal cortex and amygdalae (the mesolimbic system).

The dopaminergic system is importantly involved in signalling reward and anticipation, and salience of reward. This circuitry has evolved to signal the importance of stimuli related to survival, including hunger, thirst, and reproduction.

Drugs of addiction include diverse chemical classes with distinct targets and actions. All have been shown to increase dopamine release in the nucleus accumbens (although other transmitters, including glutamate, endogenous opioids, and norepinephrine, are involved in signalling reward). The magnitude of dopamine release induced by these drugs is much greater than that induced by conventional survival-related stimuli, which is why the motivational value of the drugs predominates over other competing motivations, and behaviour is directed towards further acquisition of the drug. The anhedonia seen in early abstinence from drugs is thought to be related to a downregulation of the dopaminergic system. The withdrawal state also increases the incentive salience of drug taking in the same way that hunger will increase the salience of food-related cues. The drug-induced changes in the motivational and reward systems are so powerful that the addicted patient will continue to use drugs when the cost of doing so, in terms of physical, psychological, social, and emotional harm, is high. Subsequently, stimuli associated with drug taking (such as specific venues and drug-taking paraphernalia) become powerfully conditioned and can trigger relapse, even after a prolonged period of abstinence.

14.5 **Drugs and the law**

Drugs that are considered dangerous to individuals or society are controlled and regulated by law. There are three international conventions under which most countries (within their own legislative framework) agree to restrict non-medical use of, and trade in, certain classes of drugs (see Box 14.4). In the UK, this legal framework (Misuse of Drugs Act 1971: the Act) applies to a number of drugs used for pain relief, including opioids, and prohibits production, supply, and possession of the drugs. For this reason, opioids are known as controlled drugs. A series of criminal offences has been established, relating to unauthorized importation, supply, possession with intent to supply, and possession of these drugs. Drugs controlled under the Misuse of Drugs Act are categorized into three classes, relating to the relative harm which they cause and the maximum penalties that can be incurred for offences against the Act (see Table 14.1).

The Regulations made under the Act define the circumstances in which specified individuals, permitted to use these drugs for legitimate purposes, may do so and specify where the drug may be produced and from whence it may be supplied. The regulations divide controlled drugs into five schedules, which relate to the degree to which their use is restricted in regard to manufacture, supply, storage, prescription, and dispensing (see Box 14.5).

Box 14.4 United Nations drug control conventions

The three major international drug control treaties are mutually supportive and complementary. An important purpose of the first two treaties is to codify internationally applicable control measures in order to ensure the availability of narcotic drugs and psychotropic substances for medical and scientific purposes, and to prevent their diversion into illicit channels. They also include general provisions on illicit trafficking and drug abuse.

Single Convention on Narcotic Drugs, 1961
This Convention recognizes that effective measures against abuse of narcotic drugs require coordinated and international action. There are two forms of intervention and control that work together. First, it seeks to limit the possession, use, trade-in, distribution, import, export, manufacture, and production of drugs exclusively to medical and scientific purposes. Second, it combats drug trafficking through international cooperation to deter and discourage drug traffickers.

Convention on Psychotropic Substances, 1971
The Convention noted, with concern, the public health and social problems resulting from the abuse of certain psychotropic substances and was determined to prevent and combat abuse of such substances and the illicit traffic which it gives rise to. The Convention established an international control system for psychotropic substances by responding to the diversification and expansion of the spectrum of drugs of abuse and introduced controls over a number of synthetic drugs, according to their abuse potential, on the one hand, and their therapeutic value on the other.

United Nations Convention against Illicit Traffic in Narcotic Drugs and Psychotropic Substances, 1988
This Convention sets out a comprehensive, effective, and operative international treaty that was directed specifically against illicit traffic and that considered various aspects of the problem as a whole, in particular, those aspects not envisaged in the existing treaties in the field of narcotic drugs and psychotropic substances. The Convention provides comprehensive measures against drug trafficking, including provisions against money laundering and the diversion of precursor chemicals. It provides for international cooperation through, for example, extradition of drug traffickers, controlled deliveries, and transfer of proceedings.

United Nations Office on Drugs and Crime. Drug Control Treaties and related Resolutions. Available from: http://www.unodc.org/unodc/en/drug_and_crime_conventions.html. Accessed May 2007.

Table 14.1 Penalties for offences of possession and supply of controlled drugs

Drug class	For possession	For supply
Class A, e.g. diamorphine (heroin), cocaine (crack), MDMA (ecstasy), lysergic acid diethylamide (LSD), and more potent opioid analgesics (e.g. methadone)	Up to 7 years imprisonment or an unlimited fine or both	Up to life imprisonment or an unlimited fine or both
Class B, e.g. cannabis, amphetamine, barbiturates, and less potent opioid analgesics (e.g. codeine)	Up to 5 years imprisonment or an unlimited fine or both	Up to 14 years imprisonment or an unlimited fine or both

Table 14.1 (Contd.)		
Drug class	For possession	For supply
Class C, e.g. cannabis, benzodiazepines (and zolpidem), ketamine, anabolic steroids, and gammahydroxybutyrate (GHB)	Up to 2 years imprisonment or an unlimited fine or both	Up to 14 years imprisonment or an unlimited fine or both

Any class B drug in injectable form is treated as class A. Some class C drugs are legal to possess, e.g. anabolic steroids are under Schedule 4 Part 2 and may be possessed in medicinal form without a prescription.

Reproduced with permission from the British Pain Society (2007). Pain and substance misuse: improving the patient experience. A consensus document for consultation. Available from: http://www.britishpainsociety.org/book_drug_misuse_main.pdf [Accessed May 2007].

Box 14.5 Examples of drugs contained in the Controlled Drugs Regulations

- **Schedule 1:** cannabis, ecstasy, LSD
- **Schedule 2:** includes opioids, such as diamorphine, morphine and methadone, and the major stimulants such as cocaine and amphetamine
- **Schedule 3:** includes buprenorphine, pentazocine, and a small number of minor stimulant drugs, such as phentermine, and some benzodiazepines such as temazepam
- **Schedule 4:** is subdivided into two parts; part 1 (CD Benz) contains most of the benzodiazepines, zolpidem, and ketamine; part 2 (CD Anab) contains the anabolic and androgenic steroids, together with five polypeptide hormones and clenbuterol
- **Schedule 5:** includes preparations of certain CDs, e.g. codeine, dihydrocodeine, morphine, that are exempt from full control when present in medicinal products of low strength.

British Pain Society (2007). Pain and substance misuse: improving the patient experience. A consensus document for consultation. Available from: http://www.britishpainsociety.org/book_misuse_patients.pdf. Ac-cessed May 2007.

There are a number of requirements relating to prescription production for Schedule 2 and 3 controlled drugs (see Appendix 1).

14.6 Risk of addiction to prescribed opioids

Exposure to reward-inducing drugs by patients using them appropriately for pain relief may result in the development of tolerance to one or more of the effects of the drug, including analgesia. Additionally, some individuals may develop physical dependence, as manifested by withdrawal symptoms following dose reduction or cessation of the drug. The majority of patients exposed to these drugs will not develop an addiction syndrome. However, the potential for opioids to be used for purposes other than pain relief (by the patient or by others) and for the development of true addiction remains a concern for prescribers. Similarly, the recognition by the patient in pain of the physical, social, and emotional decline that accompanies drug addiction acts as a barrier to accepting opioid therapy for some individuals.

14.6.1 Prevalence of addiction to prescribed opioids

The risk of developing an addiction syndrome as a result of opioid treatment for pain is not known, but there are some indicators of prevalence in the published literature. Clinical trials of opioid efficacy are too short to detect the development of a substance misuse problem. Longer-term retrospective and prospective data are available, but these need to be interpreted cautiously, as the study populations are not consistent with respect to diagnosis and previous history, and reported prevalences vary, depending on the criteria used to define addiction, including validated and unvalidated behavioural observations, DSM-III and IV criteria, Portenoy criteria, and urine toxicology.

Several prospective studies of cancer and non-cancer patients identify no substance misuse on behavioural criteria, but prevalence rates of up to 50% are also reported in one retrospective and one cross-sectional study of non-cancer pain patients. Overall, the published literature would suggest that prevalence rates from problem drug use are lower in patients with cancer-related pain.

14.6.2 Risk factors

The risk of an individual becoming addicted to opioids is influenced by genetic, environmental, social, and cultural factors as well as a number of comorbid conditions.

A family history of substance misuse is an important risk factor for addiction to prescribed drugs. The relative contributions from environmental and genetic influences within a family have been characterized by family, twin, and adoption studies, which suggest that heritability for opioid dependence is high. Genetic vulnerability is probably related to a combination of a number of 'risk genes', and the genetic risk of dependence susceptibility to one substance correlates with that for other substances, including alcohol and tobacco.

The degree to which environmental and cultural influences predispose to an increased likelihood of addiction cannot be measured accurately. Important factors are likely to include social class, occupation, and education as well as cultural perceptions (and legislation) relating to substance misuse.

A current or previous history of other substance misuse (including alcohol and nicotine) predisposes to problem drug use in relation to prescribed opioids. Non-substance misuse psychiatric disorders are also common in the substance-misusing population with lifetime rates of psychiatric disorders estimated at greater than 40%. The commonest diagnoses are personality disorders, depression, and anxiety. These disorders may increase the risk of development of a substance misuse problem, as sufferers may use psychoactive substances to alleviate unpleasant experiences. Additionally, an independent relationship between substance misuse and other mental illness has been demonstrated, suggesting that both groups of disorder may be different manifestations of a common neurobiological abnormality, possibly relating to the mesolimbic dopamine system.

Despite the consistent identification of risk factors for problematic use, prescription rates for opioids to treat non-cancer pain are much higher and increasing faster in patients with a history of substance misuse or mental health disorder. Patients with these comorbidities present some of the most formidable challenges in providing safe and effective opioid therapy.

14.6.3 **Predicting problems**

It is not possible to identify with certainty which individuals are at risk of developing problems relating to opioid use. Careful assessment is key, and there may be pointers in the history, or suggestive findings on examination or laboratory testing. Specific screening instruments for addiction and urine toxicology screening may add further information.

Clinical history

A detailed medical, family, social, and occupational history from the patient, including an assessment of their beliefs regarding their presenting complaint and their expectations regarding the outcome of the consultation, underpins any pain management plan. Patients should be treated courteously and non-judgementally and be helped to understand the importance of the accuracy of the information that they supply. Health care professionals outside the field of substance misuse may be reluctant to ask questions relating to drug-taking habits; however, patients will readily understand the importance of gathering a full picture of all substances prescribed or otherwise (including alcohol and tobacco) when they understand that it is important to support the safe prescribing of medications for pain relief. Similarly, open discussion of the relevance of identifying potential substance misuse habits amongst family and household members should support collection of this information. Patients may be concerned that disclosure of a past or current substance misuse problem, either personally or in a family member, will preclude the prescription of controlled drugs for pain relief. Patients should be reassured that therapeutic decisions will be made on the basis of clinical need and evidence of efficacy. Additional information serves to support the mutually agreed plan regarding appropriate monitoring and assessment of therapy.

It is useful to take note of concerns regarding substance misuse expressed by other health care professionals with whom the patient has come into contact. Interpretation of this information should be influenced by an understanding of why relationships with professionals may not previously have gone well for the patient. It may be useful to explore these relationships from the patient's perspective. The management of persistent pain must also be influenced by those with whom the patient is in regular contact, and it is useful to involve the patient's family or carer in the assessment.

Clinical examination

Signs of current intoxication with, or withdrawal from, alcohol or opioids may be obvious in the clinic and, if present, should be discussed with the patient. A more detailed examination may reveal signs of chronic alcohol use or signs suggestive of previous or current intravenous drug use. Routine laboratory tests (liver function tests, full blood count, and tests for infective sequelae of intravenous drug use) may corroborate the clinical impression.

There are no characteristics of a patient with a history of substance misuse that are pathognomonic, but some features of the presentation, which may support a diagnosis of substance misuse, have been described (see Box 14.6). A worrisome pattern of behaviour is unlikely to be identified on the patient's first visit but may emerge on subsequent visits.

> Box 14.6 Features of clinical presentation which may support a diagnosis of substance misuse
>
> - Current intoxication/withdrawal
> - Assertive personality, often demanding immediate action
> - May show unusual knowledge of controlled substances
> - Gives medical history with textbook symptoms, or gives evasive or vague answers to questions regarding medical history
> - Reluctant or unwilling to provide reference information. May have no general practitioner
> - Will often request a specific controlled drug and is reluctant to try a different drug
> - Generally has no interest in diagnosis; fails to keep appointments for further diagnostic tests or refuses to see another practitioner for consultation
> - Cutaneous signs of drug abuse: skin tracks and related scars on the neck, axilla, groin, neck, forearm, wrist, foot, and ankle. Such marks are usually multiple, hyperpigmented, and linear. New lesions may be inflamed. Shows signs of 'pop' scars from subcutaneous injections.

British Pain Society (2007). Pain and substance misuse: improving the patient experience. A consensus document for consultation. Available from: http://www.britishpainsociety.org/book_misuse_patients.pdf. Ac-cessed May 2007.

Screening instruments for addiction

If the patient has a current diagnosis of addiction, this may need to be managed separately (by appropriately trained professionals) in parallel with ongoing pain management. Additionally, a past or current history of an addiction problem is a significant predictor of likelihood of running into problems when prescribing controlled substances for pain. A number of specialist tools are available to screen for the presence of an addictive disorder. The CAGE questionnaire (see Box 14.7) was developed to screen for alcohol misuse and has been adapted to screen for other drug use. The questionnaire is simple to administer and has been demonstrated to be both sensitive and specific as a screening tool.

The Screening Tool for Addiction Risk (STAR) questionnaire is a validated tool that has been developed to evaluate addiction problems in chronic pain patients (see Box 14.8). A number of additional tools have been developed by specialists in addiction medicine and pain medicine, which examine patterns of prescribed use and potentially aberrant behaviours. These have utility in the ongoing evaluation of the patient who has been prescribed opioids (see Section 14.6.4 Identifying problems).

> Box 14.7 CAGE questionnaire adapted to screen for drug misuse
>
> - Have you felt you ought to cut down your drinking or drug use?
> - Have people annoyed you by criticizing your drinking or drug use?
> - Have you felt bad or guilty about your drinking or drug use?
> - Have you ever had a drink or used drugs first thing in the morning to steady your nerves or to get rid of a hangover (eye opener)?

Brown, R. and Rounds, L. (1995). Conjoint screening questionnaire for alcohol and drug abuse. Wis. Med. J., 94, 135–40.

Box 14.8 The Screening Tool for Addiction Risk (STAR) questionnaire (Friedman et al. 2003)

1. Have you felt depressed or anxious over the last 6 months?
2. Have you noticed frequent mood swings over the last 6 months?
3. Are you currently employed?
4. Do you smoke cigarettes?
5. Do you feel that you smoke too much?
6. Do you drink more than three alcohol drinks/day?
7. Have you used recreational drugs during the last year?
8. Have you ever been treated in a drug or alcohol rehabilitation facility?
9. Do you get pain medicine from more than one doctor?
10. Have you been to a pain clinic before?
11. Have you visited an emergency room for pain treatment in the past year?
12. Has anyone in your family (relatives you don't live with) had problems with drug or alcohol abuse?
13. Has anyone in your household (partner, children) had problems with drug or alcohol abuse?
14. Did any family member physically or verbally abuse you when you were a child?

Reproduced with permission from Friedman, R., Li, V., and Mehrotra, D. (2003). Treating pain patients at risk: evaluation of a screening tool in opioid-treated pain patients with and without addiction. Pain Med., 4, 186–9. © John Wiley & Sons, 2003

Urine toxicology and other laboratory tests

It is helpful to document objective information regarding drug use both to help the prescriber define a sufficiently supportive treatment plan and to minimize harm to the patient. Baseline urine toxicology screening is an important tool in this regard. Patients must be assured that clinical information collected in this way is subject to the usual rules of confidentiality. It is important that the clinician liaises with the toxicology laboratory in order that samples are collected and transported appropriately, and that the results of screening are interpreted correctly.

14.6.4 **Identifying problems**

When starting opioid therapy, a plan for monitoring progress towards agreed outcome goals, adverse effects of medication, and appropriateness of use of medication should be agreed with the patient (see Chapter 10). It is important to discuss potential tolerance to the analgesic effect of drugs at the outset of therapy, although it should be made clear that a repeated pattern of dose escalation will prompt re-evaluation of the treatment plan. It is important to emphasize the need for honest discussion regarding medication needs, as the patient, who has not yet reached an adequate dose of analgesia, may be reluctant to discuss this with their clinician for fear of the prescription being reduced or curtailed.

Prescribers of opioids must be able to identify emerging addiction problems. Savage has described behaviours relating to the three components of an addiction syndrome (continued use of medications despite harm, impaired control over drug use, and drug craving), which may be observed during opioid therapy (see Box 14.9). She distinguishes between behaviours suggestive of addiction and behaviours concordant with therapeutic use of medications.

> **Box 14.9 Behaviours that may suggest addiction in opioid-treated pain patients ('looking for the four Cs')**
>
> Adverse consequences/harm due to use:
> - Intoxicated/somnolent/sedated
> - Declining activity
> - Irritable/anxious/labile mood
> - Increasing sleep disturbances
> - Increasing pain complaints
> - Increasing relationship dysfunction.
>
> Impaired control over use/compulsive use:
> - Reports lost or stolen prescriptions or medication
> - Frequent early renewal requests
> - Urgent calls or unscheduled visits
> - Abusing other drugs or alcohol
> - Cannot produce medication on request
> - Withdrawal noted at clinic visits
> - Observers report overuse or sporadic use.
>
> Preoccupation with use due to craving:
> - Frequently missed appointment unless opioid renewal expected
> - Does not try non-opioid treatments
> - Cannot tolerate most medications
> - Requests medication with high reward
> - No relief with anything else, except opioids.

Reproduced with permission from Savage, S.R. (2002). Assessment for addiction in pain-treatment settings. Clin. J. Pain., 18, S28–38. © Elsevier 2002.

A pattern of aberrant behaviours over time is more concerning than a single observation of an aberrant behaviour. Portenoy has described these behaviours and grouped them into those more or less likely to be indicative of aberrancy.

Screening tools for aberrant drug-related behaviour have been developed by specialists in pain management and addiction medicine. These include the Prescription Opiate Abuse Checklist, the Prescription Drug Use Questionnaire, and a more recent multidimensional tool the Screener and Opioid Assessment for Patients with Pain, which has utility both as a screening tool and as a means of ongoing evaluation. The Pain Medication Questionnaire asks questions relating to behaviours and attitudes regarding the use of pain medication.

Diversion
When treating pain with opioids, it is important to ensure that the prescribed dose is taken by the intended recipient. Diversion of prescribed medications may occur by patients in pain who are receiving these drugs for pain relief and also by individuals who do not have genuine symptoms but purport to do so as a means of obtaining a supply of saleable drugs.

Diversion can include:

• Transfer of prescription drugs from intended recipient to others in pain
• Unlawful transfer of prescription drugs from legitimate to illegal channels of distribution
• Theft from manufacturers or wholesalers
• Theft from pharmacies, hospitals, surgeries, veterinary practices, care homes, hospices
• 'Prescription fraud'
• Use of over-the-counter or prescription medicines to synthesize more potent drugs with a higher street value
• Use of over-the-counter medicines to augment the effect of prescribed or 'street' drugs, i.e. the sedating anti-histamines, such as cyclizine, promethazine, or diphenyhydramine, to produce a 'buzz' with methadone.

Diversion may be difficult to detect, particularly in those without symptoms who are attempting to acquire drugs for subsequent monetary gain. Urinalysis may play a role in the evaluation of diversion, but results must be interpreted with caution. If the clinician suspects that drugs are being transferred to others in pain, e.g. family members, it is often helpful to discuss the problem with the patient's family practitioner, who may be involved in the care of those to whom drugs are being diverted and who may offer support in evaluating non-prescribed drug use in these individuals.

Managing concerns
The management of worrisome behaviours is best discussed before starting opioid therapy. When concerns arise they need to be discussed openly and non-judgementally with the patient who, in turn, must be able to reflect on the rationale for those concerns. The patient should be reassured that the goal of safe and effective analgesic therapy remains pre-eminent. Modification of the plan to evaluate the progress of therapy supports this aim. In particular, an increase in the frequency of clinic visits and prescription of small quantities of drug should be discussed as a means of re-establishing a successful treatment plan. Aberrant behaviours that appear during therapy must be comprehensively assessed and documented. This latter should include an account of discussions with the patient. If a diagnosis of addiction is suspected, it is helpful to seek the help of an addiction specialist for further evaluation and, where necessary, treatment in parallel with the continuing pain management plan.

14.7 **Management of pain in the patient with a past or current history of substance misuse**

Both persistent pain and problem drug use are common. There are, however, reasons why individuals who use illicit substances may have greater than expected needs for pain:

• Compared to those who are not dependent, the presence of a drug misuse syndrome seems to worsen the experience of pain, and individuals may have previous experiences of self-medication to remove pain and psychological distress
• Drug misusers have a low tolerance of non-pharmacological interventions to achieve pain control

- By nature of their chronically relapsing condition, drug misusers have frequent episodes of intoxication and withdrawal, which may alter the intensity of the pain experience
- Virtually all forms of addiction are associated with sleep disturbance, and this is a well-established exacerbating factor in chronic pain
- Depression and anxiety are common features in addiction, and these have an important influence on the pain experience
- Drug users are more likely to suffer from accidental and non-accidental injury, and medical complications related to their drug use. This places them at high risk from physical problems that may require analgesia.

The management of persistent pain is likely to be difficult if the patient has an unrecognized current addiction problem either to illicit or prescribed drugs. When an addiction problem has been identified, specialist support in the management of addiction will be needed in parallel with the management of pain. Patients who have recognized addiction problems should have their pain taken seriously and should be offered the most appropriate therapy for their condition, including opioid drugs if indicated. It is helpful if the patient has a clear understanding of why they have pain and also of the rationale for the appropriate treatments available.

Comprehensive assessment of both pain and addiction (as described in Section 14.6 Risk of addiction to prescribed opioids) is mandatory. The importance of a full and accurate substance misuse history needs to be emphasized to the patient. The patient needs to disclose consumption of all illicit substances consumed as well as prescribed and over-the-counter medications; this is important if adverse drug interactions are to be avoided. Assessment should also include screening for common comorbid psychiatric disorders. If present, such disorders may also need specialist support if effective pain management is to be achieved.

14.7.1 **Prescribing opioids for pain relief in the addicted patient**

Drugs used to manage addiction to opioids have important implications for the prescription of opioids and other drugs for pain control. It is helpful to have up-to-date information in this regard from the patient's specialist drug team or general practitioner. Opioid substitution therapy with methadone or buprenorphine is effective in decreasing the misuse of opioids and other substances and improves adherence to treatment; it also reduces criminal activity and improves individual function. Patients receiving a long-term opioid prescription for the treatment of addiction or those currently addicted to illicit opioids will derive little analgesic effect from their regular dose. If opioids are to play a role in the management of pain, they will need to be prescribed in addition to continuing the existing prescribed regimen. For those using illicit opioids, prescribed doses must include replacement of the patient's usual opioid consumption.

The benefits of using sustained-release opioids for the management of persistent pain are particularly important when managing pain in the addicted patient. In particular, transdermal preparations have low abuse potential. The addicted patient may be reluctant to consider change to a modified-release preparation; it is helpful to explain to the patient why this may be more appropriate for the treatment of his or her symptoms, particularly if the pain is continuous. Reassurance that the dose will be reviewed and revised appropriately may address some of the patient's concerns. Prescriptions should be issued from a single source, and it may be helpful to develop links with the patient's regular pharmacist. Ideally, the patient should be reviewed frequently as the therapeutic opioid regimen is established. The quantity of prescribed drugs should be sufficient to meet requirements between clinic visits.

It is important to develop trust between the prescriber and patient, and decisions should be taken in collaboration with the patient. Therapeutic goals and the means by which these are monitored should be agreed. There should be a frank discussion regarding acceptable and unacceptable behaviour in relation to prescribed drugs. If the patient understands the importance of adherence to the prescribed regimen, he or she should agree to appropriate monitoring of the regimen, including random urine toxicology screening. If problems develop, it may be necessary to provide more restricted supplies of medication, with an increase in frequency of review. All such discussions with the patient should be documented and a copy given to the patient if necessary. This may take the form of a formal treatment contract. If the patient repeatedly violates the agreed plan despite attempts to re-establish successful therapy, it is reasonable for a clinician to discontinue the opioid prescription in a safe and compassionate manner. In these circumstances, the care of the patient will need to be transferred to another health care professional.

When the opioid regimen has been established, the prescription of controlled drugs may be devolved to the patient's primary care practitioner. It is helpful for the pain specialist and the general practitioner to reach agreement regarding the dose of opioid and frequency of prescription. Regular specialist review is important, even if prescriptions are being provided in primary care. It is also helpful for teams involved in the management of pain in the addicted patient to communicate regarding family and social issues, which may have a bearing on the pain complaint and its management.

14.7.2 **Patients recovering from addiction**

Addiction is a relapsing disorder. Both pain and anxiety can precipitate relapse, so it is important to reassure patients that their pain will be managed adequately. If a recovered addict presents with a need for pain management with opioids, the possibility of reactivation of a substance misuse problem must be seriously considered. It may be necessary to prescribe anxiolytic drugs while the pain control plan is being implemented. Patients and clinicians need to understand that drug exposure is only one component of relapse and that a careful plan for pain management, supported by expertise in addiction problems, should allow safe management of symptoms.

14.8 **Conclusion**

There is currently no certainty regarding the risks of addiction to prescribed opioid medication, or how to identify those most at risk. The problem of inducing a substance misuse problem is inevitable for those prescribing opioid drugs, but careful assessment, collaborative working, and appropriate monitoring should identify problems if they arise. The importance of a comprehensive discussion with the patient regarding problem drug use before prescribing opioids should facilitate sensitive exploration of problems should they emerge.

Managing the addicted patient with opioids can be time-consuming and emotionally demanding for the health care team. The pain management plan will fail unless built on a relationship of trust and collaboration, and creating such relationships can be difficult for both the clinician and patient. Open and honest exchange of all relevant information regarding both substance misuse and the pain problem to be treated should allow a rational, mutually acceptable and safe, and an effective therapeutic regimen to develop and to be implemented successfully.

Key Reading

Adams LL, Gatchel RJ, Robinson RC, Polatin P, Gajraj N, Deschner M et al. (2004). Development of a self-report screening instrument for assessing potential opioid medication misuse in chronic pain patients. *Journal of Pain Symptom and Management*, **27**, 440–59.

Alford DP, Compton P, and Samet JH (2006). Acute pain management for patients receiving maintenance methadone or buprenorphine therapy. *Annals of Internal Medicine*, **144**, 127–34.

American Academy of Pain Medicine, the American Pain Society, and the American Society of Addiction Medicine (2007). Consensus statement: definitions related to the use of opioids for the treatment of pain. Available from: http://www.ampainsoc.org/advocacy/opioids2.htm [Accessed May 2007].

American Psychiatric Association (1994). *Diagnostic and statistical manual of mental disorders*. 4th edn. (DSM-IV). American Psychiatric Association, Washington DC.

Ballantyne J and LaForge S (2007). Opioid dependence and addiction during opioid treatment of chronic pain. *Pain*, **129**, 235–55.

British Pain Society (2007). Pain and substance misuse: improving the patient experience. A consensus document for consultation. Available from: http://www.britishpainsociety.org/book_misuse_patients.pdf [Accessed May 2007].

Brown R and Rounds L (1995). Conjoint screening questionnaire for alcohol and drug abuse. *Wisconsin Medical Journal*, **94**, 135–40.

Butler SF, Budman SH, Fernandez KC, Houle B, Benoit C, Katz N et al. (2007). Development and validation of the Current Opioid Misuse Measure. *Pain*, **130**, 144–56.

Butler SF, Budman SH, Fernandez K, and Jamison RN (2004). Validation of a screener and opioid assessment measure for patients with chronic pain. *Pain*, **11**, 65–75.

Chabal CMD (1997). Prescription opiate abuse in chronic pain patients: clinical criteria, incidence, and predictors. *Clinical Journal of Pain*, **13**, 150–5.

Compton P, Darakjian J, and Miotto K (1998). Screening for addiction in patients with chronic pain and 'problematic' substance use: evaluation of a pilot assessment tool. *Journal of Pain Symptom and Management*, **16**, 355–63.

Edlund MJ, Steffick D, Hudson T, Harris KM, and Sullivan M (2007). Risk factors for clinically recognized opioid abuse and dependence among veterans using opioids for chronic non-cancer pain. *Pain*, **129**, 355–62.

Fishman SM and Kreis PG (2002). The opioid contract. *Clinical Journal of Pain*, **18**, S70–75.

Friedman R, Li V, and Mehrotra D (2003). Treating pain patients at risk: evaluation of a screening tool in opioid-treated pain patients with and without addiction. *Pain Medicine*, **4**, 186–9.

Højsted J and Sjøgren P (2006). Addiction to opioids in chronic pain patients: a literature review. *European Journal of Pain*, **11**, 490–518.

Home Office Statistics (2011). Drug misuse declared: findings from the 2010/11 British Crime Survey, England and Wales. Available from http://www.homeoffice.gov.uk/publications/science-research-statistics/research-statistics/crime-research/hosb1211/hosb1211?view=Binary [Accessed November 26, 2012].

Portenoy RK (1990). Chronic opioid therapy in non-malignant pain. *Journal of Pain Symptom and Management*, **5**, S46–62.

Portenoy RK (1996). Opioid therapy for chronic non-malignant pain: a review of the critical issues. *Journal of Pain Symptom and Management*, **11**, 203–17.

Savage SR (2002). Assessment for addiction in pain treatment settings. *Clinical Journal of Pain*, **18**, S28–38.

Savage SR, Joranson DE, Covington EC, Schnoll SH, Heit HA, and Gilson AM (2003). Definitions related to the medical use of opioids: evolution towards universal agreement. *Journal of Pain Symptom and Management*, **26**, 655–67.

Strain EC (2002). Assessment and treatment of comorbid psychiatric disorders in opioid-dependent patients. *Clinical Journal of Pain*, **18**, S14–27.

Turk DC, Swanson KS, and Gatchel RJ (2008). Predicting opioid misuse by chronic pain patients. A systematic review and literature synthesis. *Clinical Journal of Pain*, **24**, 497–508.

United Nations Office on Drugs and Crime. Drug Control Treaties and related Resolutions (2007). Available from: http://www.unodc.org/unodc/en/drug_and_crime_conventions.html [Accessed May 2007].

Von Korff M and Deyo RA (2004). Potent opioids for chronic musculoskeletal pain: flying blind? *Pain*, **109**, 207–9.

World Health Organization (1992). *The ICD-10 classification of mental and behavioural disorders: clinical descriptions and diagnostic guidelines.* World Health Organization, Geneva.

World Health Organization (2004). *Neuroscience of psychoactive substance use and dependence.* World Health Organization, Geneva.

Appendix 1

Misuse of drugs regulations 2001: Prescription writing requirements for controlled drug preparations specified in Schedules 2 and 3

Prescriptions for controlled drugs (CDs), which are subject to prescription requirements, must be indelible (a computer-generated prescription is acceptable, but the prescriber's signature must be handwritten), *signed* by the prescriber and *dated*, and they must specify the prescriber's *address*. The prescription must always state (except for temazepam):

- The name and address of the patient
- In the case of a preparation, the form (e.g. tablets) and, where appropriate, the strength of the preparation
- The total quantity of the preparation or the number of dose units, in both words and figures
- The dose
- The words 'for dental treatment only' if issued by a dentist.

Note. It is advised that the maximum quantity of medication that can be prescribed is a 30-day supply. The validity of Schedules 2, 3, and 4 CD prescriptions is restricted to 28 days from the date on the prescription.

(British National Formulary (2007). *Guidance on prescribing: controlled drugs prescribing.* BMJ Publishing Group and RPS Publishing, London).

Appendix 2

Table of approximate oral analgesic equivalence

Table A2.1 Approximate oral analgesic equivalence to oral morphine*		
Analgesic	Relative potency to oral morphine	Duration of action (hours)
Codeine	0.1	3–6
Dihydrocodeine	0.1	3–6
Pethidine	0.125	2–4
Tramadol	0.2	4–6
Oxycodone	1.5–2	3–4
Methadone	1 (single dose) 3–10 (repeated dose–note:variable)	8–12
Hydromorphone	7.5	4.5
Buprenorphine (sublingual)	60	6–8
Buprenorphine (transdermal)	75 75	168 (7 days) 96 (4 days)
Fentanyl (transdermal)	100–150	72 (3 days)
Tapentadol	0.2–0.7	4–6

Adapted from Twycross R, Wilcock A, Charlesworth S, and Dickman A (1998). *Palliative care formulary*, 2nd edn. Radcliffe Medical Press Ltd, Oxford.

* These ratios provide a guide only to opioid equivalences. Conversion ratios vary, depending on the existing dose of opioid (see Section 13.4.3 in Chapter 13).

Appendix 3

Approximate analgesic equivalences of transdermal opioids

Table A3.1 Transdermal opioids: approximate equivalence with oral morphine*		
Oral morphine equivalent (mg/24 hours)	Transdermal buprenorphine (mcg/hour)	Transdermal fentanyl (mcg/hour)
10	5	
15	10	
30	20	
45		12
60	35	
90	52.5	25
120	70	
180		50
270		75
360		100

* Published conversion ratios vary, and these figures are a guide only. Morphine equivalences for transdermal opioid preparations have been approximated to allow comparison with available preparations of oral morphine.

Appendix 4

Calculating the starting dose of methadone (inpatient conversion)

- Stop morphine (or other opioid) abruptly (do not taper dose progressively).
- Prescribe a dose of methadone that is 1/10 of the 24 hour oral morphine equivalent dose up to a maximum of 30 mg
- Allow the patient to take methadone dose 3-hourly prn
- On day 6, note the total daily methadone dose over the previous 2 days and convert into a regular 12-hourly dose (Note it may be useful to prescribe less than half of the total daily dose as the 12 hour dose, thus allowing the remainder of the total to be used as required).
- The patient may be discharged on day 6 if tolerating the 12-hourly methadone dose.
- Note it may take several weeks to achieve optimum distribution of the identified daily methadone requirement throughout the day, as this will depend on the temporal nature of the pain and the experience of adverse effects. Patients should be reviewed frequently during this period.

(Scheme used by author. Adapted from Twycross R, Wilcock A, Charlesworth S, and Dickman A (1998). *Palliative care formulary*. 2nd edn. Radcliffe Medical Press Ltd, Oxford.)

Index